W9-CHL-859

Buddhist Healing Touch

Buddhist Healing Touch

A SELF-CARE
PROGRAM
FOR PAIN RELIEF
AND WELLNESS

Ming-sun Yen, M.D.,
Joseph Chiang, M.D., and
Myrna L. Chen

Healing Arts Press
Rochester, Vermont

To dear Daddy
Better late than never.

Healing Arts Press
One Park Street
Rochester, Vermont 05767
www.InnerTraditions.com

Healing Arts Press is a division of Inner Traditions International

Copyright © 2001 by Myrna Louison Chen

All rights reserved. No part of this book may be reproduced or utilized in any form or by any
means, electronic or mechanical, including photocopying, recording, or by any information
storage and retrieval system, without permission in writing from the publisher.

*Note to the reader: This book is intended as an informational guide. The remedies, approaches, and
techniques described herein are meant to supplement, and not to be a substitute for, professional medical care
or treatment. They should not be used to treat a serious ailment without prior consultation
with a qualified health care professional.*

LIBRARY OF CONGRESS CATALOGING-IN-PUBLICATION DATA
Yen, Ming-sun.
Buddhist healing touch : a self-care program for pain relief and wellness / Ming-sun Yen,
Joseph Chiang, and Myrna L. Chen
p.   cm.
ISBN 0-89281-886-7
1. Health promotion—China. I. Title: Self-care program for pain relief and wellness.
II. Chiang, Joseph. III. Chen, Myrna L. IV. Title
RA 427.8.Y46 2001
613'.0951—dc21
2001016763

Illustrations by Kam Thye Chow
Printed and bound in the Canada

10   9   8   7   6   5   4   3   2   1

Text design and layout by Virginia L. Scott-Bowman
This book was typeset in Bembo with Myria and Fine Hand as the display typefaces

Contents

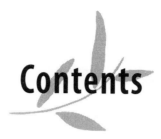

Part Three: Wellness for Life

❧

❧

Preface

This is an English adaptation of Dr. Ming-sun Yen's book written in Chinese. It is for people who mainly use the English language but are nevertheless interested in the ancient Eastern way of self-care and would like to incorporate it into their wellness routines.

Dr. Yen is a distinguished physician who has practiced medicine in Fuchow, China, for more than forty years. When he was twelve years old his family had to flee to Taiwan with the nationalist government and leave him behind. It was 1948, and the communist government took over the mainland before his family was able to send for him. The hostility between the two governments in the ensuing years affected him in a very personal way. He was not only cut off from his family and unable to rejoin them, but he was also blacklisted by the communist government because his family was working for the government on Taiwan. This "unfavorable" family background that was noted clearly on his identification papers became a source of constant hardship for Dr. Yen. He led a life of the underclass while growing up. The government even withheld his diploma when he graduated in 1958 from the University of Fuchow Medical School and barred him from practicing medicine. Because his father worked for the national government on Taiwan, Dr. Yen could not be trusted to treat patients.

After repeated protests and appeals, Dr. Yen did finally get permission to practice medicine. Unfortunately, his practice was again suspended during the Cultural Revolution in 1964. Millions of frenzied young people, mobilized by Mao Tse-tung in an attempt to crush his rivals, went on a rampage throughout the country. In Dr. Yen's city, he was an easy target of the Red Guard.

The mob condemned him; he was banished to the country for "labor reform." While serving time at the labor camp he noticed streams of people making their way up to Lin-Yang Shih, an ancient Buddhist temple on the West Mountain near Fuchow. They were seeking help from an elderly Buddhist monk. Most of the travelers had sustained physical injuries at the hands of the Red Guard. The monk treated his patients with acupressure, acupuncture, and herbs. When Dr. Yen witnessed their remarkable recoveries, he was impressed and inspired. He started to follow the monk around. For the next three years he was the monk's medical assistant. During that time the monk taught him acupressure, acupuncture, exercise, herbs, and numerous self-help methods that were handed down by his predecessors.

After the Cultural Revolution the government allowed Dr. Yen to return to his practice. At the same time, Chairman Mao was promoting the practice of healing the natural way: this was the time of the so-called Barefoot Doctor Movement. Mao believed there was no need of formal medical training—an acupuncture needle and various herbs could cure most ailments. Dr. Yen got permission from the government to incorporate what he learned from the monk into his regular practice.

While most Chinese recognize the tremendous advances that Western medicine has made, they still cling to the less invasive approach of the traditional Chinese medical practice that has existed for more than six thousand years. Dr. Yen offered the best of both worlds. His Western medical training, complemented by the traditional Chinese medicine, made him an instant success. Patients flocked to his clinic. To further his understanding of traditional Chinese medicine he enrolled at the Traditional Chinese Medical College in Fuchow, and earned a degree and a license to practice traditional Chinese medicine.

Today Dr. Yen is a leading authority on acupressure, acupuncture, and herbs. He has lectured throughout China, Taiwan, and Southeast Asia. The forty-year separation from his family came to an end when he visited his parents, three brothers, and three sisters on Taiwan. In 1989 Dr. Yen wrote this book in Chinese and had it published on Taiwan. In this book he not only included the acupressure and *ch'i kung* exercises that the monk taught him, but he also included many of the tried-and-true self-care exercises and folk cures that the Chinese have been practicing for thousands of years. Other acupressure techniques and terms as we know them today have been altered according to government guidelines to ensure political correctness. What set Dr. Yen's book apart from the many books published on this subject was the fact that he was faithful to the true tradition of acupressure that was handed down from his master, the monk.

Dr. Yen's book came to me by way of his brother Wu Tuan. He and his wife, Maria, visited us in New Hampshire and gave us the book. "The approach is easy to follow. You can use the information to cure and to prevent disease," Wu Tuan promised us. "Please share the 'good news' with as many people as you can," he urged. We read it, tried it, enjoyed it, and shared it with our many friends who read Chinese.

Another friend visiting from the Netherlands suggested an English version of this book. She told us about a nagging pain in her wrists and shoulder. My husband suggested that she try some self-help exercises in Dr. Yen's book. She tried them and they worked. Katherine wanted to know if there was an English version. "Why don't you write it in English? Think of the many people who can benefit from your work!" she said. Her suggestion was intriguing and timely.

The book became a real possibility when Dr. Joseph S. T. Chiang came into the picture. Dr. Chiang is an associate professor of anesthesiology at the University of Texas and is currently practicing at M. D. Anderson Center, ranked the top hospital in this country. He is fluent in Chinese and is credentialed to practice acupuncture. He has followed Dr. Yen's career. Best of all, he agreed to collaborate with me.

When I outlined our plan to Dr. Yen, he was ecstatic. It was his lifelong dream to have his book published in more than one language, "so many more people could benefit from this information and incorporate the self-care in their wellness routine," he wrote.

Recently, my husband and I visited Dr. Yen in Fuchow, China. Together we went to Lin-Yang Shih, where Dr. Yen met the monk healer almost three decades ago. Lin-Yang Shih is a Buddhist temple founded almost fourteen hundred years ago on the top of the West Mountain, situated on the outskirts of Fuchow. The temple is massive and magnificent, and has a panoramic view of rice fields and mountains in the distance. An auto road making the temple accessible by car is in progress. Soon tour buses will bring loads of noisy visitors to this little-known wonder of China.

We were the only visitors on that day. As dusk was approaching, the sun was setting slowly. Time seemed to stand still. The monks were quietly gathering for their evening chants. A strong sense of tranquillity, harmony, and inner peace embraced us all.

The kindly old monk has passed away. When he passed his knowledge to Dr. Yen, did he know that he had sown a very precious seed?

PART ONE

Theoretical Foundations

1 Introduction to Acupressure

This book provides an inexpensive and natural alternative to deal with our health problems and stay healthy. Instead of reaching for medicine at the slightest hint of discomfort, this book explains how to use simple acupressure on yourself to get well. We will also discuss ways to stay well by using acupressure, deep breathing, exercise, and folk cures. Most of these techniques are easy to learn, noninvasive, and can be done any-where—in the comfort of your home or away from home.

Also included are acupressure self-treatments for a wide range of specific conditions, from abdominal cramps to varicose veins. For each condition this book provides a basic understanding of the situation, the alternative treatments suggested, and what the treatments are expected to accomplish. A step-by-step guide to self-massage techniques and illustrations of the locations of the acupressure points accompany each exercise. We also look into complications that could arise and offer self-help tips. Although most topics apply to both men and women, some are dedicated to men or women only.

Traditional Chinese medicine believes that an inner energy or current of

INNER TRADITIONS

BEAR & COMPANY

HEALING · ARTS · PRESS

DESTINY BOOKS

ParkStreet Press

BINDU BOOKS

Please send us this card to receive our latest catalog.

☐ Check here if you would like to receive our catalog via e-mail.

E-mail address —————————————————————————

Name ——————————— Company ———————————

Address ——————————— Phone ———————————

City ——————— State ——— Zip ——— Country ———

Order at 1-800-246-8648 • Fax (802) 767-3726

E-mail: orders@InnerTraditions.com • Web site: www.InnerTraditions.com

Inner Traditions International, Ltd.
P.O. Box 388
Rochester, VT 05767-0388
U.S.A.

Affix
Postage
Stamp
Here

electricity known as "ch'i" regulates our health. Ch'i comes from the life "battery," the organs and endocrine glands. Out of the life battery, ch'i flows through channels called *meridians*. You can stimulate ch'i by using direct pressure with thumb or fingers on a point along a meridian, thus sending healing energy to other parts of the body. The current helps to clear carbon dioxide and toxins collected around an organ and allows the body to function more effectively. As long as ch'i flows properly, and a person's inner and outer worlds are in harmony, the body remains healthy.

The body is a wondrous machine that usually functions reliably. Occasionally, however, it requires maintenance and repair. If we learn to understand the signals of our body, we can take care of disease early on and prevent it from developing into a serious illness. Almost all diseases are related to or caused by malfunctioning organs. To treat any disease, therefore, we must first treat the affected organ.

For centuries the Chinese have used acupressure and a combination of exercises and folk cures to relieve pain and stay healthy. The methods were well documented in classical Chinese literature and books on traditional medicine. Western physicians began to pay attention to this ancient practice in the early twentieth century. In the United States, a national association for massage was founded in 1940. In 1975 there was a world conference on massage in California. In a study released for the year 1997, four out of ten Americans used alternative medicine to treat chronic conditions. Furthermore, there were more visits in 1997 to alternative medical practitioners than to conventional-care physicians. Today, acupressure and acupuncture have gained recognition and acceptance in the Western world.

There are two kinds of acupressure: passive massage, which is performed on a patient by a doctor or other trained person, and active or self-massage, in which the patient massages himself. This book is about the latter.

Self-massage is simple. You use your hands and fingers to manipulate various parts and points of your body in order to prevent illness or relieve pain. The keys to effective self-massage are correctly diagnosing the cause of the problem, properly locating the points, and accurately applying the pressure techniques.

Self-massage is easy to learn. It is noninvasive and has no side effects. By making self-massage a routine exercise, you treat a disease at the earliest stage. At the same time, you recharge your internal organs.

Most of the self-massage techniques discussed in this book can be done in your home while sitting, standing, or lying down. The only tool required is your own hands. You can even practice self-massage while working or traveling. Patience and persistence are required to make it a daily routine and a lifestyle. As long as you do not exert more pressure than you can tolerate, acupressure is safe.

Regular practice of the deep-breathing exercises described in this book will ensure proper oxygenation of all parts of your body. Proper oxygenation helps to purify your blood and remove toxins and carbon dioxide from your body. This, in turn, will reduce any unnecessary burden on your kidneys, thus minimizing the possibility of skin diseases and kidney failure. Moreover, healthy blood enables the proper functioning of all internal organs and thereby increases vitality. It will help you to stay well.

Illustrations of the locations of the acupressure points accompany each self-massage instruction. Everything is explained in simple terms rather than in medical jargon. Dr. Chiang made the necessary additions or deletions to the original Chinese version where there were conflicting medical views between East and West.

At my suggestion, Dr. Yen wrote a chapter on *gua sa* (pronounced **ga-wu-ah sa**) especially for the English version. Gua sa is a Chinese folk cure that is widely practiced throughout Asia, but has not been properly documented in English.

This book is not a substitute for your physician. Without your doctor's timely examination and diagnosis you run the risk of treating the wrong ailment. If you are pregnant or think you might be, the pressure applied to any point should be gentle; avoid pressuring the Hegu (Joined Valley), Jianjing (Shoulder Well), and Sanyinjiao (Three Yin Cross) points, and the abdominal area. Read through the exercise and discuss it with your doctor to make sure that it is safe.

Enjoy this book and share it with your friends and loved ones so all can get well and stay well.

2 How to Locate the Acupoints

To practice acupressure, first you have to locate acupoints. Your body is a road map that will show you where they are. There are various methods to locate the acupoints accurately. This book uses *cun* (pronounced tzun), also known as "the finger measurement," as the principal unit of measurement.

These measurements use a finger joint as the main starting point for measuring the length and width of various portions of the body. Each portion is one cun, a cun being the length of a midsection of your middle finger or the width of your thumb (see diagram at right). The practitioners of traditional Chinese medicine have found that the length of the midsection of a person's middle finger is a reliable measurement for that particular person.

The moveable landmarks—the clefts, depressions, wrinkles, or prominences appearing on the joints, muscles, tendons, and skin during motion—are guides for locating acupoints. For example, Chuchi (see page 6) is in the depression at the lateral end (outside) of the cubital crease when the elbow is flexed.

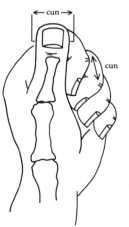

"Cun" measurement

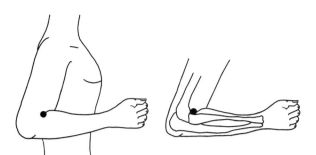

Chuchi

Each acupoint is listed in three ways in this chapter. Each acupoint is first listed in the pinyin romanization system and followed by its identification number, based on the standard set by the Administration of Traditional Chinese Medicine, People's Republic of China. The letter portion of the identification number is the meridian abbreviation, for example, LU for lung and ST for stomach. (Those that have been left blank have no identification number available.) Finally, the acupoints are listed in their original format, with Chinese characters. The literal English translations are included to give you some insight to the significance of the points.

ABBREVIATIONS OF THE FOURTEEN MERIDIANS AND EXTRA POINTS

LU—points of the Lung Meridian of Hand *(Taiyin)*

LI—points of the Large Intestine of Hand *(Yangming)*

ST—points of the Stomach Meridian of Foot *(Yangming)*

SP—points of the Spleen Meridian of Foot *(Taiyan)*

HT—points of the Heart Meridian of Hand *(Shaoyin)*

SI—points of the Small Intestine Meridian of Hand *(Taiyan)*

BL—points of the Bladder Meridian of Foot *(Taiyan)*

KI—points of the Kidney Meridian of Foot *(Shaoyin)*

PC—points of the Pericardium Meridian of Hand *(Jueyin)*

SJ—points of the Sanjiao (Triple Energizer) Meridian of Hand *(Shaoyang)*

GB—points of the Gall Bladder Meridian of Foot *(Shaoyang)*

LR—points of the Liver Meridian of Foot *(Jueyin)*

DU—points of the DU Meridian (Governor Vessel)

RN—points of the Ren Meridian (Conception Vessel)

Extra Points

> EX-HN—Head and Neck
> EX-CA—Chest and Abdomen
> EX-B—Back
> EX-UE—Upper Extremities
> EX-LE—Lower Extremities

When practicing self-masssage, one sure way to know whether you have found the specific point is that you should feel soreness, numbness, or swelling when you apply pressure to it. You may have to try several times, consulting the illustration and the description of each point.

The acupoints used throughout this book are the following.

Points on the Head and Neck

BAIHUI

DU 20 (Hundreds Meet)

On the top of the head, 5 cun directly above the midpoint of the front hairline. At the midpoint of the line connecting the tops of both ears.

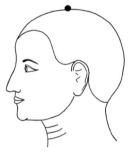

Baihui

SHENTING

DU 24 (God Court)

On the forehead, directly above the nose, 0.5 cun above the midpoint of the front hairline.

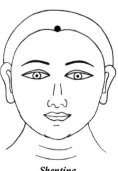

Shenting

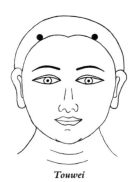

Touwei

TOUWEI

頭維

ST 8 (Head Corner)

These points are 0.5 cun above the front hairline at the two corners of the forehead, and 4.5 cun from the midline of the head.

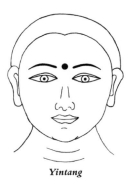

Yintang

YINTANG

印堂

EX-HN3 (Yin Court)

On the forehead, midway between the eyebrows.

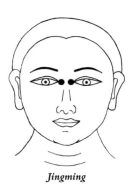

Jingming

JINGMING

睛明

BL 1 (Eyes Bright)

In the depression slightly above the inner corner of the eye.

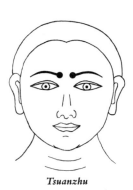

Tsuanzhu

TSUANZHU

攢竹

BL 2 (Gather Bamboos)

In the depression of the eyebrow where it meets the bridge of the nose.

YUYAO

魚腰

EX-HN 4 (Fish Waist)

In the center of the eyebrow, directly above the pupil.

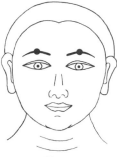

Yuyao

SIZHUKONG

絲竹空

SJ 23 (Silk Bamboo Hollow)

In the depression of the lateral end of the eyebrow.

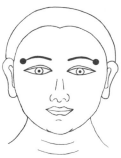

Sizhukong

TONGZILLIAO

瞳子髎

GB 1 (Eye Corner)

In the depression at the outer corner of the eye.

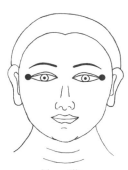

Tongzilliao

SIBAI

四白

ST 2 (Four White)

1 cun directly below the center of the pupils, on the floor of the eye socket.

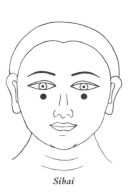

Sibai

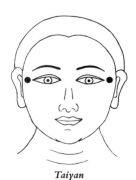

Taiyan

TAIYAN

太陽

EX-HN 5 (The Sun)

At the temple, in the depression 1 cun from the outer corner of the eye.

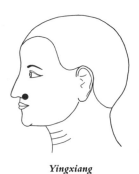

Bizuan

BIZUAN

鼻川

EX-HN 8 (Nose Stream)

Near the upper end of the nostrils, at the junction of the alar cartilage of the nose and the nasal bone.

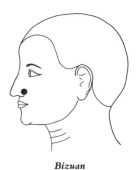

Yingxiang

YINGXIANG

迎香

LI 20 (Welcome Fragrance)

Just beyond the outer edge of the nostril.

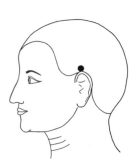

Tsewhon

TSEWHON

治昏

(Fix Faint)

Immediately above the top of the ear.

MEDIAN

米點

(Rice Point)

In front of the ear, in the depression above the upper border of the cheekbone (the zygomatic arch) where the hairline begins. Slightly higher than the Xiaguan point (see below).

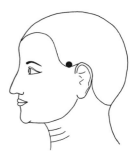

Median

TSEUDIAN

垂點

(Drop Point)

The depression immediately below the earlobe.

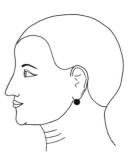

Tseudian

XIAGUAN

下關

ST 7 (Lower Gate)

In front of the ear, in the depression between the cheekbone and the lower jawbone.

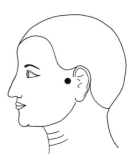

Xiaguan

JIACHE

頰車

ST 6 (Cheek Cart)

In the depression 1 cun above the jawbone.

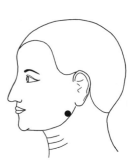

Jiache

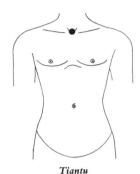

Tiantu

TIANTU

天突

RN 22 (Heaven Point)

At the front of the neck, in the hollow directly below the Adam's apple.

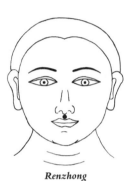

Renzhong

RENZHONG

人中

DU 26 (Person Central)

Two-thirds of the way up from the central groove of the upper lip.

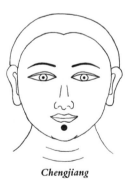

Chengjiang

CHENGJIANG

承漿

RN 24 (Receive Juice)

In the depression at the midpoint of the chin, just below the lower lip.

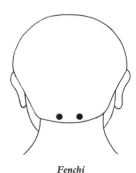

Fenchi

FENCHI

風池

GB 20 (Wind Pond)

On the nape of the neck, just below the base of the skull, in the depressions 0.5 cun lateral to the midpoint.

CHIAOGON

橋弓

ST 9 (Arched Bridge)

On the front of the neck, to the side of the Adam's apple. Located at the midpoint of the carotid artery, this acupoint feels like a rice kernel to the touch. You can feel the pulse of the carotid artery. *Caution: Never apply heavy pressure on this point or on the carotid artery.*

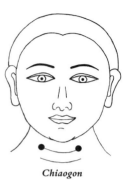

Chiaogon

Points on the Chest, Abdomen, and Waist

DANZHONG

膻中

RN 17 (Body Middle)

On the chest, midway between the nipples, on the level of the fourth intercostal space.

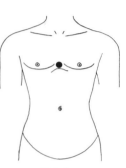

Danzhong

ZHONGWAN

中脘

RN 12 (Inner Center)

On the front midline of the upper abdomen, 4 cun above the center of the navel.

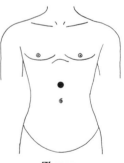

Zhongwan

SHENQUE

神闕

RN 8 (God House)

In the center of the navel.

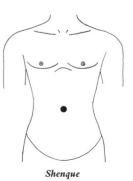

Shenque

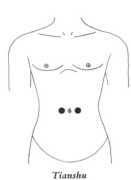

Tianshu

TIANSHU

大 樞

ST 25 (Heaven Center)

On the abdomen, 2 cun lateral to the center of the navel on both sides.

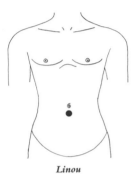

Linou

LINOU

利 尿

(Diuretic Point)

On the midline of the lower abdomen, 2.5 cun below the center of the navel.

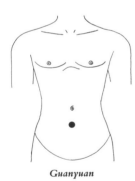

Guanyuan

GUANYUAN

關 元

RN 4 (Gate Source)

On the midline of the lower abdomen, 3 cun below the center of the navel.

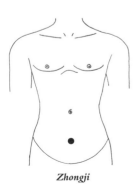

Zhongji

ZHONGJI

中 極

RN 3 (Center Most)

On the midline of the lower abdomen, 4 cun below the center of the navel.

SHENSHU

腎俞

BL 23 (Kidney Point)

On the lower back, below the second lumbar vertebra, 1.5 cun lateral to the posterior midline (at waist level).

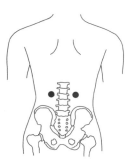

Shenshu

JIANJING

肩井

GB 21 (Shoulder Well)

On the highest point of the shoulder, directly above the nipple. This point is not recommended for pregnant women.

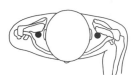

Jianjing

Points on the Upper Extremities

JIANYU

肩髃

LI 15 (Shoulder Corner)

This acupoint is in the depression in front of and below the tip of the clavicle.

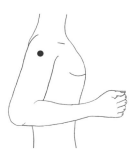

Jianyu

CHUCHI

曲池

LI 11 (Crooked Pond)

At the beginning of the elbow crease on the outside of the arm, when the elbow is flexed.

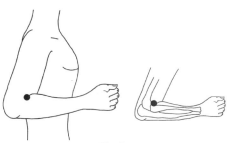

Chuchi

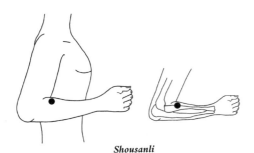

Shousanli

SHOUSANLI

手三里

LI 10 (Hand Three Mile)

On the outside of the forearm, 2 cun below the elbow crease.

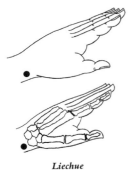

Liechue

LIECHUE

列缺

LU 7 (Line Crest)

On the radial (thumb) side of the forearm, 1.5 cun above the crease of the wrist (in the depression between the tendons of the brachioradialis and long abductor muscles of the thumb).

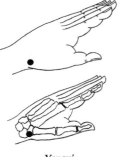

Yangxi

YANGXI

陽谿

LI 5 (Sun Valley)

At the end of the crease of the wrist, in the depression between the tendons of the short extensor and long extensor muscles of the thumb when the thumb is tilted upward.

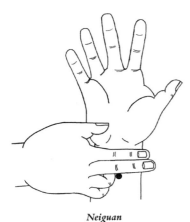

Neiguan

NEIGUAN

內關

PC 6 (Inner Gate)

On the palm side of the forearm, 2 cun above the center of the wrist crease.

SHENMEN

神門

HT 7 (God Gate)

At the end of the wrist crease below the little finger, in the depression where the hand joins the forearm.

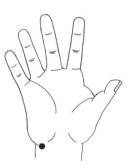

Shenmen

LAOGONG

勞宮

PC 8 (Labor House)

At the center of the palm, between the second and third metacarpal bones (but closer to the latter), in the part touched by the tip of the middle finger when a fist is made.

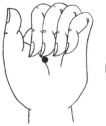
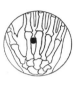

Laogong

SHAOSHENG

少商

LU 11 (Minor Sound)

On the lower outer corner of the thumbnail, 0.1 cun away from the corner of the fingernail.

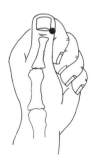

Shaosheng

SHANGYANG

商陽

LI 1 (Sound Yang)

On the lower outer corner of the index fingernail, 0.1 cun away from the corner of the fingernail.

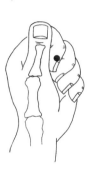

Shangyang

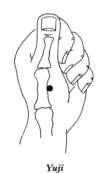

Yuji

YUJI

魚際

LU 10 (Fish Edge)

In the depression on the side of the midpoint of the first metacarpal bone (the thumb bone), at the junction of the red and white skin.

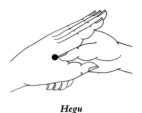
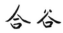

Hegu

HEGU

合谷

LI 4 (Joined Valley)

On the back of the hand in the depression between the thumb and index finger, at the highest point of the muscle when the thumb and index finger are close together. This point is not recommended for pregnant women.

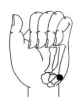

Wangu

WANGU

腕骨

SI 4 (Wrist Bone)

On the little finger side of the hand, in the depression between the base of the little finger and the triangular bone (triquetral), at the junction of the red and white skin.

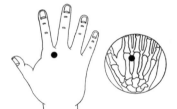
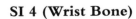

Lozhen

LOZHEN

落枕

(Drop Pillow)

On the back of the hand, between the second and third metacarpal bones.

YATONG

牙痛

(Toothache)

On the back of the hand, between the third and fourth metacarpal bones.

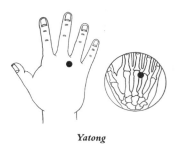

Yatong

JIAGUNG

甲根

(Fingernail Root)

This point, sometimes referred to as the matrix, is at the base of each fingernail close to the cuticle. The fingernail root can be viewed through the lunula, or half-moon, because this is where the skin of the nail is thinnest. This root point is the most sensitive part of the nail when you apply vertical cutting pressure with a fingernail of the other hand. It is a vital point, as pressure applied there can quickly alleviate the symptoms of many diseases when done correctly.

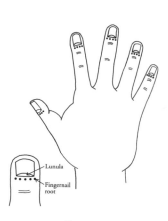

Jiagung

Use the thumbnail or the nail of the index finger of one hand to apply pressure vertically to the fingernail root of the other hand. You should feel a distinct sensation of pain. The pain and pressure applied should never be more than you can tolerate. Generally, after three to five minutes of pressure at one spot, you should begin to feel some relief. If not, move around the area and apply pressure for another three to five minutes. Each treatment can last twenty to thirty minutes. Apply pressure continuously or intermittently, depending on your tolerance of the pain and pressure.

It should be emphasized that the pressure must produce a sharp sensation of pain, and the treatment should last twenty to thirty minutes to be effective. If you stop the pressure as soon as the symptom is relieved, it may recur. Restarting the pressure may not achieve the same effect, as that particular point may become numb or its sensitivity dulled. It is therefore important to move around the point to be sure that a sharp pain is always present.

Points on the Lower Extremities

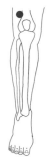

Liangchiu

LIANGCHIU

梁丘

ST 34 (Food Hill)

With the knee flexed, on the front side of the thigh and 2 cun above the kneecap.

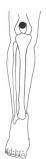

Heding

HEDING

鶴頂

EX-LE 2 (Crane Top)

In the depression in the midpoint of the upper border of the kneecap.

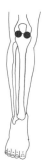

Xiyan

XIYAN

膝眼

EX-LE 5 (Knee Eye)

In the depressions on both sides of the ligaments of the knee, when the knee is flexed.

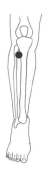

Zusanli

ZUSANLI

足三里

ST 36 (Foot Three Mile)

Below the kneecap, four finger widths (or 3 cun) below the front crest of the shinbone (tibia).

DANNANG

膽 囊

EX-LE 6 (Bile Point)

At the upper part of the outer surface of the leg, 2 cun below the depression made by the head of the tibia.

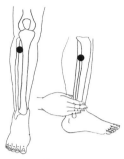

Dannang

YINLINGCHUAN

陰 陵

SP 9 (Yin Hill Fountain)

On the inside of the leg, in the depression behind and below the tip of the shinbone (tibia).

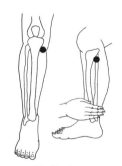

Yinlingchuan

YANGLINGCHUAN

陽 陵 泉

GB 34 (Yang Hill Fountain)

On the outside of the lower leg, in the depression below the top of the tibia (the shinbone) and in front of and below the head of the fibula (the outer and smaller of the two leg bones).

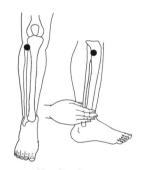

Yanglingchuan

SANYINJIAO

三 陰 交

SP 6 (Three Yin Cross)

On the inside of the leg, 3 cun (four finger widths) above the ankle, behind the inside border of the tibia. This point is not recommended for pregnant women.

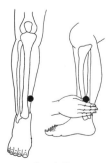

Sanyinjiao

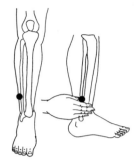

Xuanzhong

XUANZHONG

懸鐘

GB 39 (Hanging Bell)

On the outside of the leg, 3 cun above the ankle, on the front border of the fibula (the smaller of the two leg bones).

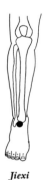

Jiexi

JIEXI

解谿

ST 41 (Relieve Valley)

In the central depression of the joint where the leg and foot meet.

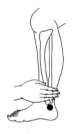

Zhaohai

ZHAOHAI

照海

KI 6 (Reflection Sea)

On the inside of the foot, in the depression below the ankle.

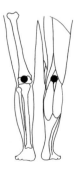

Weizhong

WEIZHONG

委中

BL 40 (Leg Middle)

At the midpoint of the popliteal crease (the back of the knee joint).

CHENGSHAN

承 山

BL 57 (Support Mountain)

On the midline of the back of the leg, in the depression below the calf muscle mass.

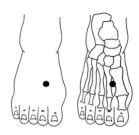

Chengshan

TAICHONG

太 冲

LR 3 (Big Gush)

In the depression between the bones of the big toe and the second toe.

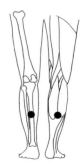

Taichong

NEITING

内 庭

ST 44 (Inner Court)

At the junction of the red and white skin near the edge of the web between the second and third toes.

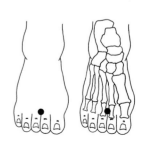

Neiting

YONGCHUAN

湧 泉

KI 1 (Rushing Well)

On the sole, about two-thirds of the way up from the heel on the line connecting the base of the second and third toes and the heel, in the depression appearing on the anterior part of the sole when the ankle is flexed.

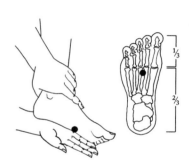

Yongchuan

3 Basic Acupressure Massage Techniques

Self-massage is done by using several different techniques. These include pressing, massaging, pushing, kneading, rubbing, moving, squeezing, patting, and cutting. The maneuvers should be gentle yet even, strong, and persistent, thereby penetrating to the corresponding organs and stimulating them.

The Techniques

Pressing

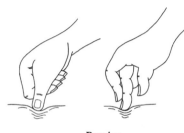

Pressing

Press with a thumb or finger vertically on the point for two minutes or less. Increase pressure gradually and keep the finger at the same spot until you feel soreness and numbness. If you feel pain, decrease the pressure gradually. It is common to rub before you press so that you can penetrate deeply into the point. Use pressing only for points on the head, fingers, or toes. If you have difficulty using your fingers, use a round-tipped pen or the eraser end of a pencil.

Massaging

With your fingers or palm on and around the point, massage in a rhythmic and gentle way. If you accidentally scrape or bump yourself, massaging in a circular motion around the wound will help prevent the wound from swelling or becoming black and blue.

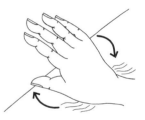

Massaging

Pushing

Move the muscle either upward or outward with your fingers or palm. The only distinct difference between massaging and pushing is the difference in pressure. You apply more pressure to pushing than to massaging. You will note that the terms *push* and *massage* are often used interchangeably in this book.

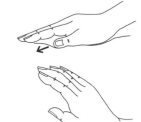

Pushing

Squeezing

Using light pressure, grasp with your hand the appropriate amount of skin, muscle, or tendon, then let go. This method is effective in treating pain and swelling of the connective tissues.

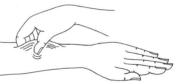

Squeezing

Kneading

Apply your hand or fingers directly on the point and move in a circular motion. Do not slide your hand or fingers over the skin. Kneading is effective in harmonizing the ch'i and blood circulation, and is good for dealing with localized pain. On the average, knead each point 80 to 120 times or for two to three minutes.

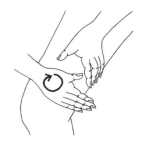

Kneading

Rubbing

With your palm or thumb closely pressed to the appropriate point, move lightly and rhythmically. Excessive force is not recommended and the rapidity should not exceed 120 times per minute. Because rubbing creates friction, the heat it produces can penetrate deeply into the area you are treating. Stop when the heat becomes unbearable. Rubbing is effective in getting rid of the cold in your body. It also enhances

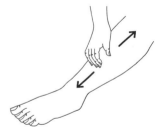

Rubbing

the smooth flow of ch'i through the meridians and increases blood circulation. When rubbing the lower back, both hands should move the same distance with the same pressure and rhythm.

Pinching

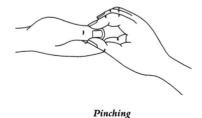

Pinching

Hold the skin or muscle of the appropriate point firmly with your fingers, then release. The intermittent exercise of holding and releasing is called pinching. Pinching is especially effective in improving the elasticity of the skin and muscle. It also improves the circulation of blood and lymph.

The difference between squeezing and pinching is that with squeezing you apply your whole hand with more force, whereas with pinching you use only fingers and thus apply less force. Squeezing and pinching often complement each other in many self-massage exercises.

Before starting any of the seven above-mentioned self-massage techniques, consider applying a coat of cold cream, gingerroot juice, or petroleum jelly on the area. This will ensure ease of maneuver and prevent the skin from inadvertent damage. You can also use tea, cooking oil, or water (boiled, if the source of water is questionable) as substitutes.

Patting

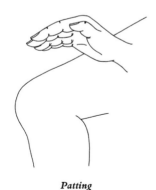

Patting

With the surface of your palm, pat the appropriate point rhythmically. Begin with light pats and increase the force and speed gradually. Start with twice per second and increase to six to eight pats per second. There should be a bounce to your movement. Most of all, you, the receiver, should feel relief with the pat.

Cutting

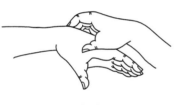

Cutting

Apply cutting pressure on the appropriate point with the thumb digging in vertically. Shake your working thumb from time to time to increase the pressure slowly and deliberately. You can also use a new, unsharpened pencil or a wooden stick that has a blunt end. It is best to cover what you use with a cotton ball or a soft tissue to avoid damaging the skin. The pressure should never be applied so forcefully that you cannot tolerate it.

Whatever methods you use, you should feel soreness, numbness, and a swelling sensation at the point being pressured.

Do's and Don'ts—Some Cautionary Notes on Acupressure

1. Your fingernails should be clean, smooth, and trimmed.
2. Make sure your palms are warm. This is especially important in cold weather. If you need to, immerse your hands in warm water or rub them together until they are warm.
3. Do not do any of the more drastic exercises when you're hungry or shortly after a full meal.
4. To reap the most benefit, first try to relax your muscles.
5. Determine the location of points with care and practice. When in doubt, read the description again.
6. Apply appropriate pressure. Do not apply excessive force on any area of your body and remember that little or no pressure will be ineffective. You should always feel some soreness, numbness, or tension in the area when treating yourself.
7. When you finish an acupressure session your body temperature will be lowered, and your resistance to cold temperatures will be lowered as well. Wear extra clothing and keep warm.

Do not perform self-acupressure or self-massage if you wear a pace maker, are pregnant, or have just had a baby. Avoid self-massage if you have a life-threatening condition such as cancer; tuberculosis; or heart, liver, or kidney disease. You should also consult your doctor if you have a serious medical problem such as an infectious disease, extensive skin lesions, acute arthritis, spinal disease, or severe stomach upset. If you are diabetic, have severe anemia, or have a disease that promotes bleeding, self-massage may not be appropriate for you. If you have just recovered from a long-term illness and are extremely thin and lethargic, you may want to give yourself some recovery time before trying any of these exercises.

PART TWO

The Practice of
Buddhist Acupressure

4 General—For Men and Women

Abdominal Cramps

Abdominal cramps are most likely caused by overeating, eating too fast, or eating food that is either too cold or too hot. To relieve abdominal cramps, try the following acupressure techniques.

- Use thumbs to apply gentle pressure to both Taichong points to relieve pain. Severe and persistent pain of the abdomen should have prompt medical attention.
- Sit or lie down and slowly press your navel (Shenque point) with your thumb. Push slowly but forcefully from your navel downward and then release. Do this twenty times. This move also relieves constipation and stomach cramps.

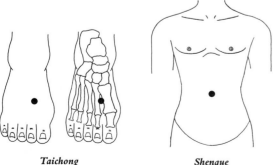

Taichong   *Shenque*

Angina

Angina, or heart pain, usually occurs in the left chest after extensive physical activity or emotional disturbance. A patient often feels nervousness accompanied by tightness, heaviness, or pressure in the chest. Sometimes the pain radiates to the jaw or left shoulder and arm. Pain usually lasts one to several minutes. It is important to rest or take the medication prescribed by your doctor. However, medication often can cause side effects such as a throbbing headache or elevated pressure in the eyes.

Generally, the best way to avoid having an angina attack is to take precautions to fend off coronary heart disease in the first place. Stop smoking, reduce your weight if you are obese, cut down the fat content in your diet, and consider doing exercise that meets the following criteria: Do the exercise at least twice weekly and for twenty minutes each time in order to strengthen your heart. During the entire twenty-minute process, the activity must maintain the heart rate at 130 beats per minute or higher. The heart rate must be no less than 180 minus your age. (For example, if you are fifty years of age, you should maintain your heart rate at 130 beats per minute or higher. If you are sixty years of age, you should maintain your heart rate at 120 beats per minute or higher.)

The exercise should involve at least 17 percent of your entire muscle mass. For example, the muscle in one arm accounts for approximately 5 percent of the muscle in the body; the muscle of one leg accounts for 20 percent; and the trunk has 43 percent of the entire muscle mass. Therefore, simply exercising both arms would involve only 10 percent of your entire muscle mass and would not be adequate.

Pick the type of exercise based on heart rate and muscle mass involved. You should also enjoy doing the exercise. Jogging, fast walking, swimming, and cross-country skiing are some suggestions. However, if you experience chest discomfort or tightness during the exercise, stop, rest, and see your physician.

The following acupressure routines may prevent angina, in some cases without side effects.

- Press and squeeze the Neiguan point of your right wrist with your left thumb or fingers for two minutes. Bend your right wrist slightly to feel and locate the exact point. Repeat with your right thumb on

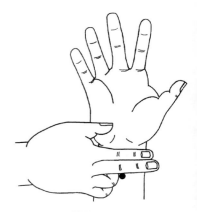

Neiguan

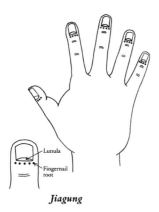

Jiagung

your left wrist. The Neiguan point should feel some pain and numbness. After applying this technique, you should feel less pressure and discomfort in the chest. Practicing this twice daily on a routine basis—once in the morning and once in the evening—can prevent angina from recurring.

- Sleep with your head higher than your feet. Ideally, the head of your mattress should be twenty to twenty-five centimeters higher than the feet. This will reduce the amount of blood return to your heart and lower the pressure on your heart. It is an effective preventive measure for an angina attack while sleeping.

- With the fingertip or nail of your right thumb, apply cutting pressure to the roots (Jiagung) of the middle and little fingernails of your left hand. Switch to the other hand and repeat. Each procedure should last three to five minutes.

Arthritic Pain in the Shoulder

Practitioners of traditional Chinese medicine theorize that when the ch'i (energy) in your body is inadequate, exterior ch'i—such as wind, cold, and dampness—will invade the body. Arthritic pain of the shoulder, therefore, has much to do with the living environment, the weather, and your physical well-being. To relieve shoulder pain and gain a full range of motion, try the following.

- For pain in the front of the shoulder, apply cutting pressure to the root point of the thumbnail on the affected side with your other thumb (see above).

- For pain on the side of the shoulder, apply cutting pressure to the root point of the fourth fingernail of the affected side with the nail tip of the second finger of the other hand.

- For shoulder pain, apply cutting pressure to the root points of the second and the little fingernails of the affected side with the nail tip of the second finger of the other hand.

In each case, apply pressure for three to five minutes at a time, twice daily. To ensure that the shoulder recovers expeditiously, you may also want to do the exercise outlined in the "Frozen Shoulder" section.

Arthritic Pain in the Knee

Knee pain can be caused by injury to the knee joint and osteoarthritis—the breakdown of cartilage in your joints. Sometimes tendonitis and bursitis can also cause pain in the knee joints. Protect your knees by staying away from peanuts, bananas, fried food, and delicacies such as sea cucumber and seaweed that are commonly found in Asian cuisine. Keep your weight down (extra weight can add extra pressure to your knees), and avoid activities that irritate your knees. Try the following exercises to relieve your pain.

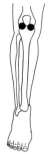

Xiyan

Liangchiu

Step 1. Sit straight in a chair. Place both middle fingers on the Xiyan points of both knees. Rub and knead for five minutes. Start gently and increase the pressure gradually, then gradually decrease the pressure. Repeat this for five minutes. While massaging, you should feel soreness or heat in that area.

Step 2. Rub and knead the following points two minutes each: Liangchiu, Zusanli, Yanglingchuan, Heding, Sanyinjiao, and Weizhong. You should feel soreness and heat while massaging.

Step 3. With both palms, rub the outside and the back of the leg. Start from the lower calf area and gradually move to the upper part of your leg. Do this twenty times.

Step 4. Tap with loose fists starting from the outside of the lower leg. Move toward the back and then upward. Do ten repetitions.

Step 5. Bend and stretch your knees gently ten times to conclude the exercise. (Avoid bending your knees at more than a 90-degree angle, however.)

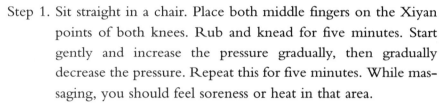

Zusanli   *Yanglingchuan*

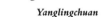

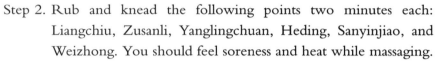

Heding   *Sanyinjiao*

- If you do the above-mentioned exercise twice daily and continue for at least six months, your knee joints should feel a definite improvement.

- This is a supplementary exercise: In an upright position, lean your upper body slightly forward. Your feet should be shoulder width apart and your knees slightly bent. Hold your knees with both hands and rotate them clockwise ten times, then counterclockwise ten times. Stand straight and rest when necessary. Repeat this exercise two to four times a day. It is important to move slowly, in as large a circle as possible.

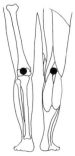

Weizhong

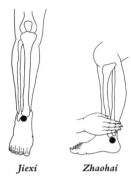

Jiexi   *Zhaohai*

- For ankle pain: Apply cutting pressure with either your thumb or second finger to the Jiexi point and Zhaohai point and where it hurts the most for two to three minutes each.

Asthma

Asthma attacks can be provoked by allergies, infections, pollutants, or changes in mood, weather, and location. You can be overcome suddenly by shortness of breath or breathing difficulties if you have asthma. In a severe attack, you may fight for breath as well as become pale and clammy, with your lips or tongue turning black and blue. In this case, call an ambulance or go to the hospital immediately.

Spasms of the airway, mucus obstructing the airway, constriction of the air passages, and oxygen deprivation are also common complaints of asthma patients. If you can manage to expel phlegm, you'll feel much relief.

Although asthma deaths have been on the rise over the past decade, this drastic result can be avoided if you know how to manage your asthma condition. Having your disease properly diagnosed and learning to manage your bronchial dilator medication will improve your quality of life. These are some of the things you can do to alleviate the symptoms of asthma.

- The best way to prevent or survive an asthma attack is to closely monitor sudden changes of weather and environment, watching out for such things as the heat and dust of a suffocating muggy day. Understand your triggers. For example, if your asthma symptoms are worse at certain times of the year, plant pollen is probably the cause. Keep your car windows closed at all times and bedroom windows closed at night. Use air-conditioning if feasible. Listen to the weather service and stay indoors when pollen counts are high. Rinse your hair before going to bed at night and do not use sheets or wear clothing that have been sun dried.
- Cut down on or eliminate tobacco use. Avoid stress and physical overexhaustion. Avoid relying too long on a drug that once helped you breathe easily. Practice the deep-breathing exercise outlined later in this section.
- Here is an exercise to help relax muscles in airways during an attack. Keep in mind, however, that this is not a cure. Massage the Danzhong point

with your fingers at the rate of twice per second, gently at first and increasing the pressure gradually. Generally, massage for three to twenty minutes depending on how long it takes to relieve your condition.

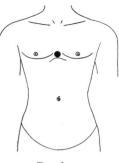

Danzhong

- Squatting is a position that can relieve your condition. It is best not to overeat while suffering the asthma attack.
- Practice deep breathing. Stand, sit, or lie down. Put one hand on your chest and the other on your abdomen. Try to inhale as much air as possible with your abdominal muscle instead of your chest. To exhale, empty all the air from the abdomen. Breathe with a regular rhythm, deeply and gently. The rate of exhaling should be two or three times slower than the rate of inhaling. Inhale through your nose and exhale through your mouth as if whistling. Breathe seven to eight times per minute. Practice this twice a day for ten to twenty minutes each time. If you do this exercise persistently, you will find that you will be able to breathe more comfortably.

Back Injury

Back injuries are common among athletes and active persons. Sudden changes of posture, accidents, or any kind of direct impact can result in a back injury. Learning the correct posture for lifting heavy objects can cut down on injuries to the back muscles, spinal vertebrae, discs, or nerves. Seek timely treatment after an injury to stave off the potential danger of sustaining long-term back pain.

According to the degree of injury and location of the injury, select the exercises that best suit your situation.

- Lie on your abdomen, preferably on a hard surface or a board. Place the base of your right palm (or thumb) on the waist where pain is most prominent. Place your left palm on the back of your right hand. Breathe deeply. While exhaling, push both hands downward forcefully. While inhaling, lift both hands. Repeat this exercise five or six times. This exercise is effective when you have twisted and injured the muscles around the waist.
- Stand with knees bent and feet shoulder width apart. If necessary, hold on to a steady object such as a chair or a countertop. Breathe deeply. While

inhaling, bend your knees as low as you are able but keep your back straight. While exhaling, rise to a standing position. Do five or six repetitions, then bend and abruptly stand up. Repeat this more abrupt movement five or six times. This exercise is effective for an injured lower back.

- Here is an acupressure exercise. Before you attempt this, you will need to pinpoint where the pain is most prominent. If is is located predominantly at the centerline of your back, it is associated with the Du Mo or Governor Vessel Meridian. If pain comes from both sides of the centerline, it is associated with the Taiyan Gin or Sun Meridian.

    In the case of Du Mo, apply pressure on the Renzhong point with the tip of your thumb or index finger. Rub the point in a circular fashion and you should feel soreness and swelling. Apply pressure for three to five minutes.

    In the case of Taiyan Gin, if the pain is to the left of the center, apply pressure on the right Wangu point, and vice versa. Press the Wangu point with the tip of your thumb, moving in a clockwise direction for three to five minutes. You should feel soreness and a swelling sensation. Some people feel relief after only one session, others may need several sessions and should press the Renzhong (see above) and Weizhong points for an additional minute.

    If you can not readily identify the exact location of the pain, press both the Renzhong and Wangu points. The sooner you take action to relieve your pain, the more effective these methods will be. However, if after repeated sessions the pain worsens or radiates downward, stop the exercise. Seek the help of a doctor immediately.

- When you sustain a back muscle injury, try resting on a bed with a hard board under the mattress, or on a bed with a mattress that fits the contour of your back.
- Stand erect. Slowly bend your upper body forward and then backward. Then bend to the left and to the right. Do this exercise as often as you like.
- After recovery from the initial injury, exercise to strengthen your back muscles. In the beginning, the exercise should be slow and gentle. As time goes on, increase the rate as well as the rigor of the exercise.

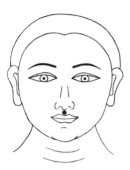

Renzhong

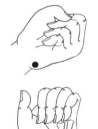

Wangu

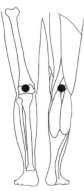

Weizhong

Back Pain

Backache is not an illness in itself but a clinical manifestation of various other ailments. It can be brought on by spinal conditions, neurological disorders, and kidney disease. In pregnancy, it may be a warning sign of either a miscarriage or the onset of labor. Fractured or broken bones and discs can also cause acute back pain. It is therefore important to consult a physician for proper diagnosis and treatment. Although the etiology of back pain is complex and varied, statistically 90 percent of back pain falls into two major categories—the overstretched and injured back muscle and arthritic back pain.

Generally, pain is located at both sides of the back where the major muscle groups are. It can also be limited to one side or to the middle—the centerline of the back. After prolonged sitting, standing, walking, overexertion, or strenuous exercise, the pain gets worse. It should diminish after adequate rest. When stretching and bending, you will feel a pulling sensation in the back muscle. There is usually an obvious pressure point that is sensitive to the touch. The muscle may be so tense that there are knots that are hard to the touch. In some cases, the back is immobile and affects your sleeping and eating routine. Some people eventually develop chronic arthritic back pain.

Arthritic back pain moves around the body. Traditional Chinese medicine believes that it is affected by prolonged living in cold and damp conditions or camping on damp grounds. Patients with arthritic backache tend to like warm and dry climates. Even strong wind can be bothersome to them. The body movement becomes quite rigid. Back pain can be a weather barometer because weather changes may be associated with the onset of back pain.

Although a great majority of patients suffering back pain fall into the above two categories, there is no breakthrough medication that can completely cure them. Our movements such as walking, carrying heavy burdens, or bending forward, backward, and sideways all rely on our back muscles. It behooves us to avoid heavy and improper lifting and to exercise to keep the muscles toned, especially if there was previous back muscle injury.

The following three back muscle strengthening exercises offer several approaches. Give each a try and pick one or a combination.

This first one is a series of massage techinques.

Step 1. With both hands on your waist, and thumbs pressed hard on the Shen-

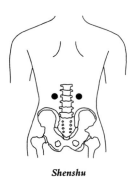

Shenshu

shu points, rub both points in a circular movement for ten minutes. If there is an area on the back where you feel soreness or pain to the touch, rub it with the thumb for ten minutes. Begin the rubbing with light pressure and gradually increase the pressure to the extent that you can tolerate it. If your fingers get tired from the massage, rest and then resume. After extended and regular massage, you may be able to loosen or minimize the knot since you are increasing the circulation to that area.

Step 2. Tap both sides of the waist evenly with loose fists for two minutes.

Step 3. In a standing position, bend your waist forward, backward, and then turn left and right. Exercise for two minutes.

Step 4. Rub both palms together until they are nice and warm. Then rub the back muscles in an up and down motion slowly and deliberately until you feel warmth in the back area. If you suffer from arthritic back pain, rub twice daily for as long as you are able to.

Traditional Chinese doctors believe that the back muscles protect the kidneys. Kidneys prefer warmth and not cold. Rubbing improves circulation and keeps the kidneys warm. When the kidneys are healthy, the body's overall health is enhanced. Therefore, traditional Chinese doctors often approach back pain by first improving the well-being of the kidneys. They often recommend the use of a hot water bottle or heating pad on the back to relieve pain and bring warmth to the back muscle area.

- The first exercise is known as the Flying Swallow. This exercise is more suitable for middle-aged persons. Lie flat on your stomach on the floor or on a board with arms at the sides of your body. Raise your arms, legs, and head upward at the same time, like a flying swallow. Try to hold that position for five to ten seconds, and then return to the original position. Do not bend any other joints and keep your chest on the floor or board. Practice this three times daily, each time for ten minutes.

- This next exercise, known as the Arched Bridge, is more suitable for the elderly. Lie flat on your back on a hard surface. Place a pillow under your waist and then add another, so that your body is arched like a bridge. Do this exercise two or three times daily, each time for twenty minutes.

- Walking backward. Pick a level path with few pedestrians and no traffic. The ideal time for this exercise is in the morning when the air is fresh.

Walk backward for four to five hundred yards and increase the distance gradually. The speed and length of the walk can be varied. Look back from time to time in order not to trip and fall. Keep your legs straight. Breathe evenly. You can either throw your hands to the sides or hit your back muscles with your fists while walking backward.

This is a technique developed by the Japanese. It is popular in Japan because it has been found to increase the elasticity of the back muscles and stabilize the spine. Walking backward uses the thigh muscles rather than the smaller calf and buttocks muscles. It decreases the impact on the kneecaps, thus permitting you to exercise without irritating any inflamed areas. Many also have claimed that the pain has subsided or even disappeared as a result.

If you have chronic back pain, avoid sudden twisting of the waist and any overexertion. Keep your back warm, and be mindful of proper sitting and standing postures. Sleep in a bed with a board underneath a firm mattress that fits the contour of your back.

Calf Cramp

Although some people experience uncontrollable muscle contractions during the day, most people suffer muscle spasms in the middle of the night. You wake up with excruciating pain and a spasm in the feet or legs. The contraction of the muscle makes it hard and tense. At times, the big toe points upward or sideways while the rest of the toes move involuntarily.

Cramps can be vascular or muscular in nature. Women suffer vascular cramps that are usually brought on by varicose veins, pregnancy, and thrombophlebitis (inflammation of a superficial vein). The muscular cramp usually occurs after high-impact exercise such as running, swimming, and long-distance cycling. Some of the known conditions that cause muscle spasms are extreme cold weather, unaccustomed exercise, pregnancy, calcium deficiency, and impaired blood flow to the leg muscles. To prevent muscle spasms, massage and stretch your muscles properly before any high-impact exercise. Keep your feet warm to avoid sudden muscle spasms while sleeping. Consult your physician to rule out the possibility of thrombophlebitis and deep-vein thrombosis.

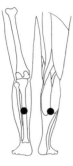

Chengshan

In the case of a sudden muscle spasm, do any of the following exercises.

- Stand with both feet on the ground. Pull the upper part or the big toe of the afflicted foot toward you, or push that part of your foot against the floor.
- Stand with both feet closely aligned. Place your hands on your kneecaps. Plant both heels firmly on the ground and lean your upper body slightly forward. This should stop the muscle spasm immediately.
- Apply heavy pressure on the Chengshan point with your finger. This should relieve the cramp gradually.

Cervical Spinal Diseases

Cervical osteoarthritis—arthritis of the neck bones—is common in people more than sixty years of age. It is also more prevalent among people who routinely work behind a desk and bend their necks while doing their work—a watch repairman who does precision work, for example. If you lead a sedentary life, you are also more prone to suffer from this. If you jolted your neck and think you may have damaged the spinal cord, consult a physician as soon as possible.

Patients who have spinal disease often complain of a crackling sound with neck movement and frequent neck pain and stiffness in the morning. Neck pain can be continuous or intermittent and often radiates to the head, shoulders, arms, and fingers, which can feel cold, numb, and heavy. Sometimes the pain is excruciating, with stabbing or burning sensations that often affect the patient's ability to work and sleep. In the worst situation, patients occasionally faint.

To prevent or minimize such problems, try these techniques.

- Sit or stand and move your head from one side to the other, like the pendulum of a clock. In the beginning, do this exercise a few times in the morning and again in the evening. You can do this while looking out the window or watching television. You may feel dizzy from moving left to right in the beginning. As you get used to the exercise, you can move as many as one to three hundred times per session.

This is also helpful to people with high blood pressure because neck exercise improves blood circulation and blood supply to the head and strengthens the neck structure that supports the head. Prolonged and regular exercise can reverse the protruding cervical spine disc, thereby relieving pressure on the nerve root.

- In daily life, pay attention to maintaining the stability of your spine at the neck. It is best to take preventive measures rather than seek remedial treatment. Some pointers are as follows.

> Do not turn your head suddenly on hearing unexpected noise.
>
> Sleep on a medium-soft pillow. If you must read in bed, place the book at a 45-degree angle.
>
> If you've been sitting for a long time, take a break to stretch every now and then. Stand up and massage both sides of your neck and shoulders to ensure that blood is circulating properly.
>
> When the weather turns cold, protect your neck and shoulders with a muffler or scarf. If necessary, apply a heating pad on your neck prior to going to bed to relieve your aches and pains.

Cold Sores

For people who reside in colder regions, cold sores and frostbite that recur yearly can be a nuisance. Here are preventive measures that you can use. Combined with normal care, this should cure the cold sore once and for all.

Beginning in the fall or before the cold weather actually hits, until the end of the next spring, maintain the following regimen.

- Massage the old wound with your palm or fingers vigorously for five minutes, or until the area feels warm.
- Increase or continue your daily physical exercise to build up your resistance to the eventual cold weather.
- Keep wounded areas dry. Stay away from the cold wind if the wounded area is wet.
- Keep the wounded area warm. For example, wear a muffler, gloves, warm socks, and so on.

- Apply an ice cube to the area as soon as you feel a cold sore coming on. This may prevent the cold sore from developing. Avoid direct skin contact with others.

Colds

Common colds usually happen during a change of season, most notably the onset of spring, fall, or winter. Sometimes following exposure to cold and wet weather conditions, your upper respiratory tract suffers a catarrhal disorder. It is often marked by headaches, lethargy, fever, coughing, sneezing, runny nose, and general indisposition. It is important to take precautionary measures to avoid catching a cold or the flu if you're more advanced in age. With old age, colds are often followed by serious health-threatening complications.

Following are various suggestions to care for the common cold.

SELF-MASSAGE

This is a useful exercise to ward off a cold if done daily. Do it in a room with no draft and drink some hot broth or eat some hot cereal before this exercise.

Step 1. In a yoga position, sit on the floor or a mat with your legs crossed and tucked under your body. Rub your palms vigorously until they are very warm, then place one hand on your forehead and rub the back of your neck with the other hand one hundred times. Switch hands and repeat one hundred times.

Step 2. Clasp the back of your neck with both hands and push your head forward until your chin touches your chest. Do this one hundred times.

Step 3. If you begin to perspire after step 2, close your eyes and concentrate your thoughts on the area two fingers below your navel—the Dantien—for about fifteen minutes.

HEAT MASSAGE

Step 1. Push the Fenchi points with your thumb and index finger for two minutes.

Step 2. If your temperature is over 100°F, push hard on the Chuchi points on both arms for two minutes with your thumb or index finger.

Step 3. If aches and pains accompany a cold, rub the Shousanli point on both arms for two minutes each.

Step 4. Place a hot wet towel over both ears for ten minutes. Chinese medicine considers that ears are closely related to the internal organs. The ears will send the warmth throughout the system when they are stimulated by high temperatures. Apply a hot towel twice daily, including once before bedtime.

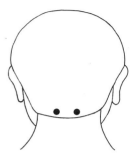

Fenchi

STEAM

Use a humidifier or vaporizer in your bedroom. Make sure the steam is not too hot. You may want to add slices of gingerroot or chunks of garlic to the water. If you have a stuffy nose and find it difficult to breathe through your nose, inhale the steam through your mouth.

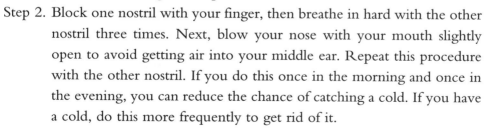

Chuchi

WATER STIMULATION

Step 1. Fill a basin with warm water. Use your hands to scoop up some water, hold it in front of your nose, breathe it into your nostrils, and then let it flow out. Take care not to let the water get into your throat. If you have access to a nasal cup, place the spout of the cup in one nostril and pour water through it. Repeat this three to five times for both nostrils.

Step 2. Block one nostril with your finger, then breathe in hard with the other nostril three times. Next, blow your nose with your mouth slightly open to avoid getting air into your middle ear. Repeat this procedure with the other nostril. If you do this once in the morning and once in the evening, you can reduce the chance of catching a cold. If you have a cold, do this more frequently to get rid of it.

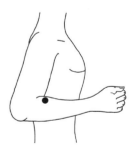

Shousanli

Step 3. Fill a bowl with warm water. Immerse your face, blinking your eyes and blowing your nose for ten seconds.

Water can help to clear clogged passages and prevent buildup of irritants that lead to colds. Not only can it decrease common colds and flu, but it can also reduce minor headaches and sometimes improve sleep.

Constipation

Guh Hung, a Chinese medical expert during the Jing dynasty, had a famous saying: "If you want to live long, leave your stomach often empty. If you do not want to die, keep your intestine often empty." He was essentially saying that the secret to a long and healthy life is to eat less and have regular bowel movements.

There is no substitute for consuming plenty of water and high-fiber foods such as fruits, vegetables, and unrefined cereals. Stay away from spicy food, coffee, and tea. Exercise regularly, breathe with your abdomen, and never put off defecation when you feel the urge.

Scientists nowadays pretty much agree that constipation can cause side effects such as lack of appetite, bloating, and indigestion. In the case of an elderly person with hypertension, constipation may trigger a stroke.

The following exercises can help you deal with constipation.

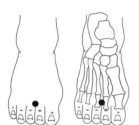

Neiting

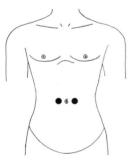

Tianshu

- If constipation is a rare occurrence, you can press the Neiting points of both feet with your thumbs for three to five minutes. It is best to do this in the morning before your bowel movement.
- If constipation is habitual, try this exercise. Lie on your back and bend both legs. Place your palm on your abdomen and move counterclockwise around the navel sixty times. Now move clockwise with the other hand for sixty rounds. Do this once in the morning and again in the evening. Your movement should be steady yet gentle. In most cases, constipation will disappear after fifteen days of practicing this exercise.
- When defecating, you can also apply pressure with the left index finger on the right Tianshu point located about 2 cun from the navel. When you feel a distinct sensation of soreness, keep pressuring that spot. You should have a bowel movement in ten to twenty seconds. If this doesn't work the first time, try again. It will work eventually.

Coughing

Coughing is a mechanical defensive reaction that helps to expel foreign objects and phlegm in the throat. To cough properly and get rid of phlegm, try these techniques.

- Take a deep breath and then press the Tiantu point with your finger. This will build up inner pressure that will help get rid of phlegm. This method is especially useful for patients with chronic lung disease.
- Inhale slowly and deliberately through your nose and exhale with your mouth in a whistling motion. Then open your mouth, stick out your tongue, and cough. If you've just had surgery and coughing is painful, place a pillow on the sutures.
- Buddhist monks often practice the following exercise. If you suffer from chronic bronchitis, you should use this one frequently.

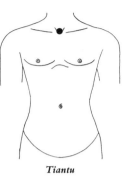

Tiantu

Step 1. Sit on the side of a bed with your feet planted on the floor. Make fists with both hands. Try to lift your buttocks with your fists and feet, then lower your body onto the bed.

Step 2. Still sitting on your bed, bend your upper body forward. Reach and grab the tips of your toes with your hands, then let go. Repeat this three times.

    Repeat both steps twenty-four times. Then close your eyes and sit quietly for fifteen minutes.

Dandruff

If you have dandruff—excessive flaking and itching of the scalp—avoid fattening foods and sweets. Eat lots of vegetables and foods with a high vitamin B content. When shampooing, apply a moderate amount of antidandruff shampoo and lukewarm water. Try the following exercise.

- Massage your scalp with your palms for ten minutes. Do this twice every day. Dandruff will usually disappear in a week or so. After the dandruff disappears, massage once every other day.

Diabetes

Diabetes often manifests the "Three Too's" in patients—eat too much, drink too much, and urinate too often. Over time, the patient becomes thin and lethargic.

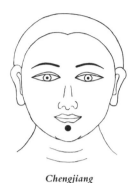

Chengjiang

With proper diet, medication, and the following exercises, you can achieve amazing results.

- Tightly squeeze the Chengjiang point and the surrounding area ten times with the tips of your fingers. Do this two to three times daily. You'll feel saliva gushing out, thus lessening the constant thirst. This movement helps to relieve the dry-mouth syndrome that is a common diabetic complaint and to adjust the metabolism of the body.
- Lie on your back and relax your entire body. Place all your weight on your head and heels (do not bend your knees), and suspend your body in a bow shape for as long as you can. In the beginning, you may need the help of your arms to elevate your body. Do this three to five times each session and twice daily.

Diarrhea

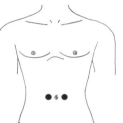

Tianshu

Diarrhea—frequent and watery bowel movements, sometimes uncontrollable—is caused by indigestion, spoiled food, allergic reactions to food, and cold, heatstroke, and certain drugs. If you are suffering from diarrhea, limit your intake of fruits and juices but drink more water to prevent dehydration. If you are vomiting, take fluids in small, frequent sips. Consult with your doctor to rule out the possibility of serious disease.

In most cases, the following self-massage exercises will help.

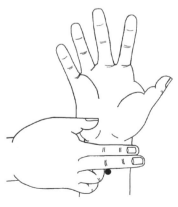

Neiguan

- Lie on your back and press your navel and the two Tianshu points (one on either side of the navel) with your thumbs and two middle fingers. Rotate all three points simultaneously for three to five minutes.
- If you are vomiting along with the diarrhea, press the Neiguan point of your right wrist with your left thumb for two minutes. Bend your right wrist slightly in order to feel and locate the exact point. You should experience some numbness and pain. Do the same with your left wrist.

Difficulty Swallowing

If you have difficulty swallowing, or vomit immediately after ingesting food, try the following.

- This exercise is best done in a gym and with an empty or nearly empty stomach. Grab the rings or bars, suspending your feet and body off the ground. Breathe lightly several times. Move your feet back and forth eighteen times in the air.

    Then sit down and close your eyes. Move your tongue up, down, left, and right until the saliva begins to fill you mouth. Swallow the saliva. Do this two to three times. *Note:* This exercise is also suitable for patients diagnosed with esophageal cancer in the early stage.

Difficulty Walking Due to Aging

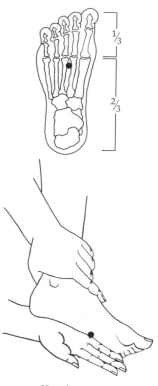

Yongchuan

According to a Japanese newspaper, an institute for the aged in Japan developed an exercise for the elderly who have trouble walking. After practicing the exercise, many started to walk again without the assistance of a cane, and some elderly who were confined to wheelchairs started to walk along the wall. This exercise was introduced to patients in China. Based on Dr. Yen's experience, eight out of ten patients were able to walk on their own after they did this exercise consistently.

Although good for the elderly, this exercise can be used by any person as a preventive measure.

- Massage your toes. Grab each toe with your hand and rotate it, starting with the little toe. Do this on both feet, fifteen minutes each. Stretch both legs afterward.
- Tap the bottoms of your feet. Tap the Yongchuan point with a small wooden or plastic hammer for ten minutes each, twice daily. If in the beginning you find it difficult to do this exercise yourself, try to find someone to help you with the exercise.

Dizziness, Faintness

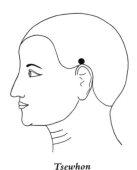

Tsewhon

Dizziness and feeling faint are common symptoms that could be triggered by any of the following: cold, flu, insomnia, anemia (iron-poor blood), hypertension, hypotension, low blood sugar, severe air pollution, and poor health. Blurred vision may accompany the dizziness in some instances. The symptoms will go away if you stand or sit still with your eyes closed. In more severe cases, you will feel nauseated, experience vomiting, or even faint.

Select one or more of the following treatments.

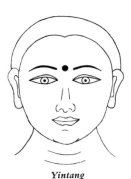

Yintang

- Press the index fingers tightly on the Tsewhon, or Fix Faint, points located immediately above the apex of the earlobes. Close your eyes and move both fingers back and forth across the points thirty-six times (in about thirty seconds). If the dizziness seems serious, increase the movements to one hundred times. You should be able to see and think clearly after the massage. Repeat two to three times daily.
- Press the Yintang point with the entire nail surface of the middle finger for one to two minutes, until your forehead feels sore and swollen. To make it more effective, you may also want to press the Renzhong point and Baihui point for one to two minutes each.
- Lie on your back, bend and raise your leg, and shake it a few times. Then bend and straighten your leg in a kicking motion a few times. Do the same with the other leg.
- Grab your wrist with the other hand and twist it back and forth fifteen times. Do the same with the other wrist. (This exercise can only treat mild dizziness, however.)

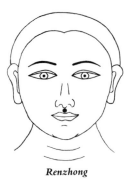

Renzhong

Emphysema

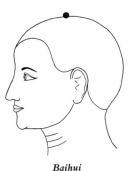

Baihui

Emphysema is a chronic degenerative lung disease often caused by the loss of elasticity of the alveoli. Breathing becomes difficult and shortness of breath occurs.

You can increase your breathing capacity by practicing this deep-breathing method regularly.

- Stand, sit, or lie down. Put one hand on your chest and the other on your abdomen. Try to inhale as much air as possible by expanding your abdominal muscles instead of your chest. When exhaling, contract the abdomen and expel all the air. Breathe with an even rhythm, deeply and gently. The rate of exhaling should be two or three times slower than the rate of inhaling. Inhale though your nose and exhale though your mouth in a whistling motion. Breathe seven to eight times per minute. Practice this twice a day for ten to twenty minutes each time. If you do this exercise persistently, you will find that you will be able to breathe more comfortably.

Enlarged Abdomen—The Beer Belly Syndrome

We all know that a beer belly is made of abdominal fat and not beer. It affects not only your appearance and your movement, but also your overall well-being.

Whenever possible, massage and pinch the abdomen where there is a thick accumulation of fat with your thumb and index fingers. The following is a good preventive exercise.

Step 1. Do the deep-breathing exercise at least three times daily and do thirty repetitions each time. See the directions for this exercise under "Emphysema."

Step 2. Stand up and interlock your hands at the back of your head. Twist your upper body from side to side.

Step 3. Lie down on the floor, placing both palms and heels firmly on the floor. Raise your abdomen off the floor and then lower it.

Step 4. Sit on the floor and bend your knees. Hold on to your knees and try lifting your feet off the floor. Balance yourself with only your buttocks touching the floor, then extend your legs forward slowly with both heels on the floor. At the same time, swing your arms backward. The motion of your body is similar to rowing.

Practice steps 2 through 4 at least twice daily. Repeat as often as time and energy allow and increase the frequency as time goes by. Strengthening the abdominal muscles, you will cause the beer belly to slowly disappear.

Eye Strain

You may feel faint and dizzy after working long hours with your eyes. Words become blurred and objects double. These are symptoms to warn you that you have probably overworked your eyes.

The following techniques for massage and rest can help alleviate the symptoms.

- Either stand or sit, keeping your head and upper body erect. Roll your eyeballs clockwise and then counterclockwise, slowly and deliberately, eight times.

  Look to the left and then to the right, eight times each way. The sweep should be swift with a pendulum-like rhythm.

  Look up as far as you can until you can see the dark edge of your own eyelid, then look down as far as you can. Repeat this movement sixteen times.

  Rub both palms until they are warm, then close your eyes and cover them with your palms for a few minutes. Then look out the window.
- If you feel sleepy and tired but need to stay awake, sit up straight in a chair and pull both shoulders back. Hold your chin up and drop both hands so that your palms are perpendicular to the seat cushion. Tighten your back, hand, and neck muscles for ten to twelve seconds and then relax.

If none of these exercises works, it's time to take a rest.

Foreign Object Lodged in the Windpipe (The Heimlich Maneuver)

Should some food or foreign object become lodged in your windpipe, stay calm. Try coughing up the object if you can. Your first choice is always to get assistance and medical help. Try using the Heimlich maneuver on yourself if there is no one available to assist you.

- Use your fist (with the thumb inside), or the back of a chair, or a table against your stomach above the navel and below the rib cage. Swiftly and forcefully, thrust in an upward and inward motion against your stomach. Repeat until the object is dislodged. The theory is that the outside force on your abdomen reduces the capacity of the chest cavity and forces the air in the lungs to rush upward through the throat, thereby ejecting the foreign object.

Familiarize yourself with this maneuver now rather than wait for an emergency and have to read the directions for its use. Time is of the essence.

Frozen Shoulder ("The Fiftieth Shoulder")

If you did not have your shoulder checked out and cared for after an injury, years later it may reappear as "frozen shoulder." This is due to bands of scar tissue that form between the ball of the humerus and the shoulder socket, thus limiting the shoulder's range of motion. Long-term overuse of the shoulder muscle can also cause frozen shoulder. Frozen shoulder usually preys on the elderly and the weak since their blood circulation is generally under par and their shoulder joints and surrounding muscles have atrophied. The medical term for this condition is *adhesive capsulitis*. Chinese doctors call it "fiftieth shoulder" because most patients are more than fifty years of age.

People who suffer from frozen shoulder experience pain and stiffness that worsens at night. Some patients cannot put on their own clothing, or wash themselves, comb their own hair, or eat by themselves. In the worst case, the shoulder is locked in place and cannot perform any simple movements. If you allow the symptoms to go on for a long period of time without treatment, the muscles of the affected area, being inactive, will also atrophy and lead to further limitation of movement.

The massage and exercise outlined below will improve the blood circulation, thereby improving the well-being of the shoulder muscle. They will also slow down the atrophying of the muscles. Once the pain has disappeared, it normally does not recur.

Step 1. In a sitting position, try to raise your affected arm to shoulder level with your thumb pointing upward. The Jianyu point is the hollow inden-

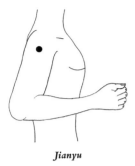

Jianyu

tation at the highest point of the shoulder. Press it with your index or middle finger and bring the affected arm down slowly at the same time. Continue to press the Jianyu point for two minutes.

Step 2. In a standing position, rub your affected shoulder to relax the muscle. Then swing that arm from front to back and left to right. Increase the speed from thirty times per minute to eighty times per minute and widen the angle gradually. Do this exercise for ten minutes, twice daily. The ideal place for this exercise is outdoors in fresh air. Initially, you may have to help lift the affected arm with your good arm or get someone to help you.

Raise the hand of your affected arm above your head. Slowly try to touch the opposite shoulder by coming down over your head.

Place the hand of your affected arm on the back of your head and try to touch the shoulder blade on the other side.

Place both hands on the bottom of a wall. Climb the wall with both hands to as high as you can reach, then slowly climb down to where you started. Repeat this twenty to thirty times and practice it twice daily.

Stand erect or sit straight in a chair. Make a loose fist with the opposite hand and pat your affected shoulder one hundred times.

Gallstones

The excruciating pain caused by gallstones often happens to obese persons in their late fifties. It frequently occurs in the middle of the night. When that happens, you are awakened by continuous dull pain. The pain usually spreads from under your ribs on the right side of your abdomen. As the pain worsens, it often radiates to your right shoulder or to your back. At times, you may also feel nauseated and vomit.

Do the following exercises to alleviate the pain, and try to get to a hospital as soon as possible.

- Press the Dannang (bile) point on your right leg with the right thumb or middle finger. The Dannang point is located about 2 cun below the depression made by the tips of your leg bones, and is very sensitive. Press it lightly at first, then apply as much pressure as you can tolerate for two minutes.

- Press the Zusanli points on both legs with thumbs or index fingers for three to five minutes. This will help alleviate the pain caused by the gallstones.
- Apply a hot compress on your upper right abdomen for thirty minutes.

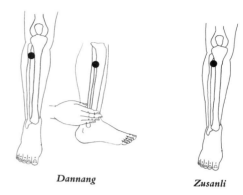

Dannang   *Zusanli*

Gastroptosis—Downward Displacement of the Stomach

Gastroptosis is the medical term for the downward displacement of the stomach. Patients with gastroptosis often become uncomfortable after eating. (This can be relieved by lying down.) At times patients feel nauseated, vomit, suffer slight stomach cramps, and lose their appetites. The situation is exacerbated by a reduced intake of food, lethargy, palpitations, fainting spells, and constipation alternating with diarrhea.

In order to control this illness, you must first think positively, and follow a routine lifestyle—early to bed and early to rise, for example. Eat small amounts but eat often, and plan your diet carefully to ensure that foods are nutritious and easy to digest. Rest appropriately after each meal, ideally for one hour. Exercise on a regular basis.

In addition, do the following exercises.

- This first exercise is a massage technique called "ring around the abdomen." Lie on your back and relax your stomach muscles. Using the navel as the center point, massage clockwise with your palm one hundred times. Repeat with the other hand counterclockwise one hundred times. The pressure should be firm yet gentle. This will enormously improve the blood circulation of your digestive system.
- Stretch both arms forward and sit up while holding your breath. Then lie down and rest for thirty seconds. Do as many repetitions of this sit-up as

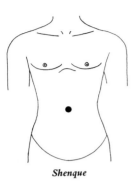

Shenque

you can. In the beginning, you may only be able to practice it for a few minutes. Increase the duration gradually until you have reached the ten-minute goal.

- Sit or lie down, and slowly press your navel (Shenque point) with your thumb. Push slowly but forcefully from your navel downward, then gradually release. Do this twenty times.

Do these three exercises once in the morning and once in the evening. During the day, in your spare time, stretch and bend your waist to strengthen your stomach muscles.

Note: Always consult a doctor for proper diagnosis and treatment. After the situation is under control, use these exercises as rehabilitative measures.

Gum Disease and Tooth Decay

Approximately 50 percent of middle-aged people suffer varying degrees of periodontal disease. Periodontal disease destroys the bony structure of the tooth. Eventually the tooth becomes loose and falls out. Self-massage can improve circulation in the gums and strengthen the bones of the teeth. Prior to practicing this self-massage, have a periodontist do a thorough checkup and cleaning to remove any plaque.

There is no substitute for frequent brushing, flossing, and rinsing after you eat to prevent tooth decay and gum disease. Avoid sugary foods because bacteria acts on sugar to produce acids that attack the tooth's protective layer. Interestingly, the World Health Organization considers tooth decay along with heart disease and cancer as the three preventable diseases.

The following massage will improve blood circulation in the gum tissues and help prevent the development of gum disease.

- Wash your hands. Then massage the gum with the full length of your index or middle finger in a horizontal direction, working upward for the upper teeth and downward for the lower teeth. Massage the gum for each and every tooth thoroughly. Massage the left quadrant of the gums with the right hand and vice versa. The massage takes ten to fifteen minutes and is best performed after brushing your teeth. Also, consider using an electric toothbrush and gum massager. The ideal time to do these massages is after thoroughly brushing and rinsing your teeth in the morning and evening. Brushing, flossing, and rinsing after each meal, combined with massaging your gums twice daily will keep gum disease and tooth decay under control.

Headaches

In our daily lives we often encounter many "headaches." In order to solve them we knit our brows while searching for answers. When you frown your neck muscle contracts, restricting blood flow to that muscle, and causing muscle pain. When you try to work out a problem, you think intensely and your brain has to work especially hard. Eventually dizziness, ringing in the ears, and real headaches occur.

Also called a muscle-contraction headache or stress headache, the tension headache is the most common ailment of all. The following self-massage methods not only combat tension headaches, but also alleviate colds, heatstroke, and insomnia.

- When you feel pain in your forehead, press your Shenting, Yintang, Tsuanzhu, and Yuyao points, in that order. Then press the Taiyan and Sizhukong points.
- When the pain is in the temples, press the Taiyan and Sizhukong and Touwei points. If you have a cold and a headache, press the Fenchi points as well.

Press the points for at least one to two minutes, using both

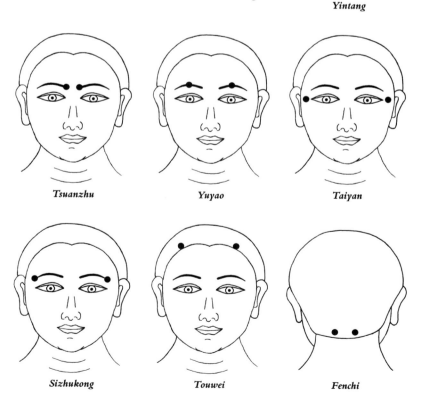

Shenting

Yintang

Tsuanzhu

Yuyao

Taiyan

Sizhukong

Touwei

Fenchi

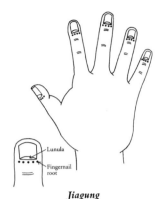

Jiagung

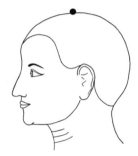

Baihui

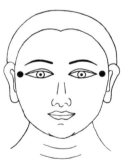

Taiyan

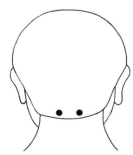

Fenchi

hands when appropriate, and apply enough pressure to induce soreness and numbness. Breathe deeply while pressing.

- Also press the fingernail roots (Jiagung).

    For a frontal headache, apply a cutting pressure to the root of your index fingernail, first on the left and then on the right for three to five minutes.

    For a migraine headache, press the roots of both your ring fingernails. If the migraine headache affects only one side, just press the root of the ring fingernail of the affected side.

    If the headache is concentrated more on the top of your head or the back of your neck, apply a cutting pressure to the roots of both fingernails of the little fingers.

    Press the root of the fingernail with the fingernail of the other hand at a 90-degree angle, hard enough to cause distinct but tolerable pain. In normal circumstances, you should feel relief after three to five minutes. If not, you can gradually move your pressure point lower and repeat for three to five minutes.

- Patients with hypertension often complain of dizziness and headaches. To relieve headaches, wash your hair with warm water. Use your fingertips to massage the Baihui point, both of the Taiyan points, and both of the Fenchi points.

    If the headache extends to your neck, grab your neck between the Fenchi points with the four fingers together and the thumb on the other side. Knead ten to twenty times.

Your head, eyes, and neck should feel instant relief after the exercise. Repeat the massage once in the morning and once at night for one week. This should alleviate the headaches considerably. The combination of massaging with fingers and warm water stimulates the nerve endings, improves the circulation, and relaxes the many nerves in the face and head.

Some headache-related danger signs that you should be aware of are:

sudden and severe headache with no warning signs
headaches lasting one week and getting worse as days go by
headaches accompanied by convulsions

headaches accompanied by a decreased sense of touch

headaches while sleeping or, worse, waking up with a violent headache

headaches worsened by coughing or stretching

headaches accompanied by a high temperature and stiff neck

a violent headache during the third trimester of pregnancy

a headache accompanied by dizziness, vomiting, distorted vision, confusion, or loss of speech, especially if these symptoms follow a recent blow or injury to the head

the sudden onset of a severe headache in a normally healthy elderly person (in this case, consult a physician immediately)

Heart Palpitations

Under normal conditions, most people have a heart rate of sixty to eighty beats per minute. Only when you are agitated, excited, or exhausted do you experience an increased heart rate and shortness of breath. After a rest, the heart rate and breathing will return to normal. Heart palpitations, however, can occur when you're sitting quietly, lying down, or even in your sleep. Your heart pounds and you suffer a period of rapid heartbeat.

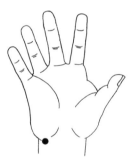

Shenmen

If the palpitations are caused by a heart condition, they have the potential of being life threatening. You should consult a doctor to rule out heart disease. Palpitations can also be caused by nervousness, agitation, insomnia, heavy smoking, drinking, overeating, and too much coffee or tea. Think back and try to understand what actually caused the palpitations.

When the doctor has ruled out a heart condition as a possible cause, pick one or more of the following ways to alleviate the symptoms.

- With the fingers of the left hand, press and pinch the Shenmen and Neiguan points of your right hand for two minutes each. Do the same on the other hand.
- With the tip of your right thumb or index finger, press the root (Jiagung) of the middle or little fingernails of the left hand for three to five minutes. Do the same on the other hand.
- When you sense palpitations coming on, drink some water or eat

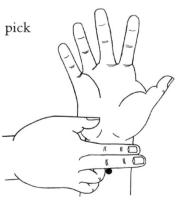

Neiguan

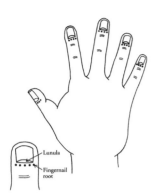

Lunula
Fingernail
root

Jiagung

some fruit. Find someone to talk to or listen to music. When you divert your attention, palpitations often diminish or disappear altogether.

• Often you can slow down your heart rate by taking a deep breath, holding it for a few seconds, then exhaling deeply and slowly. Or you can start by exhaling deeply, holding your breath, and then inhaling deeply and slowly.

Hemorrhoids

Hemorrhoids may be internal or external. Many people who have them are symptomless, or have only occasional, brief bleeding. If you see blood on your toilet tissue or notice changes in your bowel patterns, it is important to report this to your physician to rule out any possibility of a serious underlying disorder such as gastrointestinal disease, including cancer.

There are no sure ways to prevent hemorrhoids. But you should eat a high-fiber diet, avoid constipation, wear cotton underwear and loose clothing, get regular exercise, and try not to strain just because you think you have to have a good bowel movement daily or always at a set time. Do not delay if you feel the urge to have a bowel movement. Do not use the toilet seat as a reading chair; it will only encourage swelling. Do not lift heavy objects. Keep the anal area clean and use soft tissue to avoid irritation.

Sun Si-yuan, the great medical authority during the Tang dynasty, stated in his thesis on wellness that to "exercise the rectal function regularly" is one of the sixteen ways to stay healthy. Patients with hemorrhoids have found the following exercise helpful. You can also use it as a preventive measure because doing this exercise regularly may help to avoid constipation, prolapse of the uterus, and prostate cancer.

• Close your mouth, clench your teeth, push your tongue toward the roof of your mouth, and contract the sphincter muscle upward and inward as tightly as you can. Hold this position for a count of five. Then slowly let go. Practice this forty to fifty times and repeat the exercise four times daily. Ideally, practice it once in the morning, once in the evening, and before and after a bowel movement.
• Sit in a bathtub of warm water.

- Apply cotton pads soaked in an astringent such as witch hazel on the affected area.
- Cold compresses also may bring relief.

Hiccups

Hiccups are often caused by improper eating. Sometimes they're caused by severe nerve disease or chronic deterioration of the kidney functions. Hiccups usually last only a few minutes, but if they persist for a whole day or even longer, they can be very painful and exhausting. Hiccups sometimes precede serious illness and should not be ignored. If they persist for two days and none of the remedies works, consult a doctor.

Every ethnic group and culture have remedies for hiccups. China is no exception. Try the following.

- Plug both ears tightly with your little fingers for five minutes.
- Close your eyes and gently massage your eyeballs with your index fingers. You should feel some tolerable pain. Massage twice daily, two to three minutes each time, until the hiccups stop completely.
- When you're hiccuping, think of a complicated, hard-to-solve problem you are facing. Or try calculating a math problem, reciting a poem, recalling an incident from the past, and so on. Before you know it, the hiccups are gone.
- Induce sneezing by inserting a feather or cotton swab into your nostril and moving it around. The hiccups will go away when you sneeze.

High Blood Pressure

Generally, blood pressure varies with age. Most people's blood pressure fluctuates. Hypertension can be related to long-term stress, lack of physical activity, and heredity. It can also be brought on by kidney disease. We will discuss only the former type of hypertension.

The following therapeutic exercises are designed to deal with various symptoms of mild to severe high blood pressure.

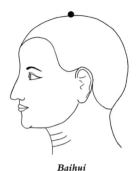

Baihui

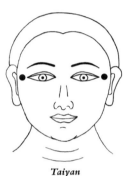

Taiyan

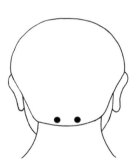

Fenchi

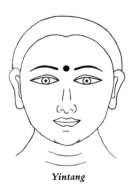

Yintang

- When your blood pressure is above normal, dizziness and headaches are two common complaints. To relieve headaches, wash your hair daily with warm water. With your fingertips, massage the Baihui point, both of the Taiyan points, and both of the Fenchi points in the back of your neck. If the headache extends to your neck, grab your neck between the Fenchi points with four fingers together and the thumb on the other side. Rub ten to twenty times. Your head, eyes, and neck should feel instant relief after the exercise. Repeating the exercise once in the morning and once in the evening for one week should alleviate your headaches. The combination of warm water and massaging your head stimulates the nerve endings, improves the circulation, and relaxes the many nerves in the face and head.

- If your hypertension has reached the acute stage—the diastolic maintains at 130 or above consistently—wash your hair while taking a shower. You may also ask someone else to wash your hair for you. Sit on a chair that will allow you to lean backward and tilt your head.

    Try not to lean forward. The person assisting you should be gentle and his or her movements evenly distributed while washing your hair.

- The following self-massages are recommended for those of you who do not have any symptoms of hypertension or whose hypertension is in the early stage. Generally, blood pressure fluctuates in the early stage. When you are stressed, agitated, overworked, and exhausted, your blood pressure rises. After resting, blood pressure returns to normal. Try these simple exercises.

    "Dry clean" your hair. Sit in a chair and run your fingers through your hair from front to back ten times.

    Rub your forehead. Sit in a chair and, using the length of the entire index finger of both hands (the sides close to the thumb), rub from the Yintang point to the Taiyan points (see above) ten times.

    Massage the upper extremities. Stand or sit. Rub the left arm from the shoulder down to the back of the left hand with your right hand ten times. Repeat on the right arm.

    Abdominal massaging. Lie on your back and remove any restraints such as a belt. Using the navel as the center, massage the abdomen with one hand clockwise for two minutes.

With the other hand, massage the abdomen counterclockwise for another two minutes. If you do this exercise regularly, it will help lower your blood pressure and improve your digestion.

Deep breathing. Stand or sit. Place both palms on your chest. Inhale through your nose, exhale through your mouth. While exhaling, move both hands slowly and gently from your chest to the lower abdomen. Repeat three times.

Massage the lower extremities. Sit and place your right hand on the inner side of the upper left thigh and your left hand on the outer side of the left thigh. With both hands, slowly massage downward toward the back of your left foot. Repeat ten times. Then switch to the right leg and repeat ten times.

Foot rub. Sit and rub both hands until the palms are very warm. With your right palm rub the sole of your left foot vigorously until the foot feels warm (approximately two hundred times). Always rub the Yongchuan point (Rushing Well). Repeat the same on your right foot. Frequent foot rubbing can clear the vital systems of your body, help you to sleep better, clear your throat, and improve your eyesight. In addition, it will help relieve nausea and a stuffy nose.

Soaking your feet in warm water before doing the foot rub will enhance these effects.

Follow the above sequence and perform the massages once in the morning and once in the evening. You should notice some improvement in your blood pressure in a week.

The relaxing exercise. Sit in a chair or sit in the lotus position, preferably in a quiet room or corner of the house. Concentrate on the center portion of your lower abdomen (the Dantien). Do your best to block out noise and sight in your mind. Stare blankly and calm yourself completely. Repeat the word "relax" to yourself. Sense your body relaxing and feel the blood and ch'i flowing downward. In the beginning, practice this for thirty minutes, twice daily. If possible, increase the exercise to three to four times daily. The main

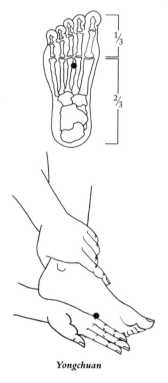

Yongchuan

purpose is to bring the blood and ch'i to your lower body. Relax completely and breathe normally. If you have trouble breathing normally, cannot concentrate, or feel agitated, you should stop the exercise. Otherwise you will cause the blood pressure to rise. If you can achieve the main purpose of the exercise, you will become very adept at it after a month or two.

If you find the relaxing exercise difficult, replace it with the relax reflex method. A quiet and peaceful environment and a comfortable posture (sitting or reclining) are two requisites. Repeat a single word or phrase when you exhale. Try to block out anything that is bothering you.

If your hypertension is more advanced, you will need to control it with medicine. Only after the blood pressure is under control should you start the above-mentioned exercise. It is effective but the effects are too slow to be immediately noticeable. Besides self-massage, methods such as the relaxing technique; outdoor exercise such as walking, biking, swimming, and jogging; controlling your weight; and eliminating or limiting sodium, caffeine, alcohol, and tobacco from your diet are also recommended. Eat more food with vinegar and calcium. Go to bed and get up at a regular times. Maintain a happy mood and balance your daily activities. These are all good preventive measures.

• When their blood pressure rises, most people tend to resort to their medication immediately. If you apply your fingers to the Chiaogon point and move from the top of the neck slowly and gently downward, you can lower your blood pressure. The Chiaogon points are located on the sides of the neck on the carotid artery, close to the Adam's apple. When your blood pressure rises, the Chiaogon point will feel hard like a small pebble and will vibrate strongly to the touch. Move the hard point gently downward but never apply heavy pressure. As the blood pressure lowers, the hardness should disappear. This exercise will not only bring the pressure down quickly, but can also slow a rapid heartbeat.

Another quick and easy way to prevent your blood pressure from ri-

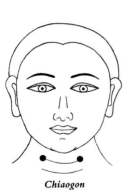

Chiaogon

ing when you feel agitated or excited is to repeat the deep-breathing method ten times. Breathe in quickly and breathe out slowly and deliberately. Refer to the deep-breathing method outlined under the section devoted to asthma.

Indigestion

People with chronic indigestion often feel bloated, stuffed, and uncomfortable after eating. Although there are many preparations available over the counter, it's better to learn to eat slowly and allow yourself half an hour of relaxation after a large meal.

Try the following exercises to alleviate indigestion.

- Rub the center of your left palm with your right thumb fifty times. Repeat this on the right hand. Do this exercise three times daily for fifteen days.
- With one hand on the other, push and massage your stomach area (underneath the left rib cage) in a circular motion from left to right fifty times. Practice this exercise once in the morning and once in the evening; it will help increase your appetite.
- You may want to add thirty minutes of slow walking after each meal to improve digestion. Since a healthy digestive system is the key to a healthy life, even if you have never had indigestion, you may want to do this as a preventive measure.
- Lie on your back and relax your abdominal muscles. Using the navel, or Shenque point, as the center of your circle, massage clockwise with your palm one hundred times. Then alternate hands and massage counterclockwise for one hundred times. The pressure should be strong yet gentle.

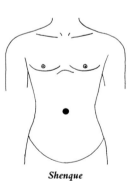

Shenque

Insomnia

How much sleep do you need? If you are like most people, about eight hours a night is an adequate amount. However, some need at least nine and yet others are totally refreshed after a routine six hours per night. Sleep experts believe genetics probably play a role. Occasional sleepless nights caused by specific incidents are normal. However, persistent and prolonged sleeplessness is a problem. Worse, insomnia is often accompanied by headaches, dizziness, heart palpitations, forgetfulness, ringing in the ears, and lethargy during the day.

Insomnia can be caused by many factors. Emotional stress such as depression, anxiety, unexpected setback, difficult or unresolved problems, sadness, worry, extreme excitement, and anticipation of an event account for most chronic insomnias. Physical illness and certain medications can often disturb sleep. Poor sleeping habits such as watching late-night television and sleeping in can confuse your body's normal sleep and wake cycles.

Insomnia isn't an illness and it's not difficult to overcome. The key is to regulate your mind and daily habits.

- Before going to bed, deal with your problems by writing down your worries and possible solutions. You may not be able to solve a problem, but decide on at least one step you can take.
- Avoid novels, movies, and television programs that provoke too much excitement.
- Stay away from spicy food, caffeine, alcohol, and nicotine that can keep you from falling asleep or cause you to wake up often.
- Engage in vigorous exercise daily.
- If your days are stressful or hurried, relax for a while before bedtime.
- Boredom can also cause insomnia. Look for new challenges that enrich your life.

Medication can alleviate the symptoms of insomnia but can't cure the cause. Here are a few ways to combat insomnia without taking sleeping pills.

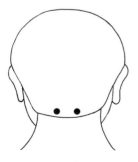

Fenchi

- Every evening before going to sleep, vigorously rub your right Fenchi point with your right index finger and your left Fenchi point with your left index finger for four to five minutes. Do this for five days.
- This is a ch'i kung exercise. Lie down and place your hands on both sides of your navel. Cross your left foot over your right. Lightly touch the roof

of the mouth with the tip of the tongue. Concentrate your thoughts on the lower abdominal area. Breathe normally and naturally. Your feet will slowly become numb, a sign that you're falling asleep.

- Get under the covers as if you're going to sleep. Move your head gently from the center to the left about 10 degrees and roll it back in one or two seconds. Count the back-and-forth movements silently from one to one hundred, then count from one to one hundred again. Do not pay too much attention to the counting. As you move your head, you can reduce the angle of movement from 10 degrees to 9 and then 8. This is similar to the movement of a cradle that gradually decreases as the infant appears to fall asleep.

- Lie on your back and tap your upper teeth with your lower teeth twice per second while counting silently from one to one hundred, then start from one again. The tapping speed does not have to coincide with the silent counting. Don't worry if you have miscounted or lost count. Simply continue to count or start counting again. This exercise is especially effective for curing insomnia due to mental overwork or stress.

- Use a fragrance you find pleasing or place an apple next to your bed. Establish a relaxing bedtime ritual such as reading, listening to soft music, or knitting.

- It is also helpful to eat a light dinner. Never eat before going to bed (this also helps you to maintain your weight). If you need something before retiring, drink a glass of water. Water has no calories but it sends a message to your brain that something has just been ingested, thereby relieving your hunger. If you still feel hungry, eat light and easily digestible food.

- The great scholar of the Sung dynasty, Master Su Tung-poh, devised a four-part method to combat insomnia. Massage, proper posture, relaxation, and routine are his four teachings.

Before going to bed, massage the Yongchuan points on the soles of the feet, two hundred times for each foot. This will not only allow you to fall asleep more easily, but also to sleep more soundly. Nowadays traditional Chinese doctors further recommend that you soak your feet in very warm water until your whole body feels the warmth, then massage the

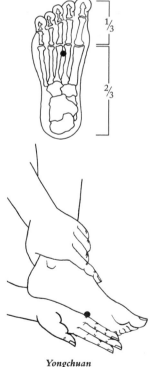

Yongchuan

Yongchuan points.

The proper sleeping posture, according to Master Su, is to lie on your left side, bending the right leg at the knee and keeping the left leg straight. This posture can protect your heart from pressure as well as prevent nightmares. Relax your body; try not think of unpleasant or trivial things; breathe normally.

The fourth teaching of Master Su is routine. By that he means go to bed and get up at a set time every day.

Involuntary Blinking

Involuntary twitching of the eyelids is caused by nervousness, overwork, or insufficient rest. When your eyelids contract involuntarily, it is irritating. The more you're irritated by the jumpiness, the more your eyelids twitch. It's a vicious cycle. Normally your eyelids will stop twitching as soon as you get proper rest. But if they do not stop, here are some easy massage techniques that should help.

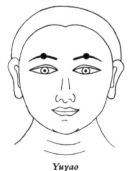

- For the upper eyelid, press and rub the Yuyao point.
- For the outer corner of the eye, press and rub the Tongzilliao point.
- For the lower eyelid, press and rub the Sibai point.

In each case you need to press and rub for one to two minutes with your index finger. Then press the Hegu point of the affected side for one minute.

If you massage directly on the eyelids where the contractions occur, you may accomplish the same result.

Yuyao

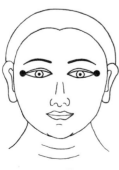

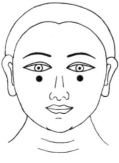

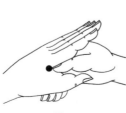

Tongzilliao   *Sibai*   *Hegu*

Migraine Headaches

Migraine headaches are triggered by sudden blood flow changes to the visual cortex of the brain. The blood vessels in the brain and the meninges (membranes that envelop the brain) dilate and cause surrounding tissues to swell painfully. Typically, a migraine manifests on one side of the head and is often accompanied by nausea, vomiting, and hypersensitivity to light and sound.

Since the etiology of the migraine is not totally known, we focus our treatment on preventing flare-ups and alleviating them when they do occur. If you have recurrent headaches, keep a diary of when they occur. Note the food, medication, situation, and anything that may be associated with the migraine attack. You or your doctor may be able to figure out what is triggering your headaches.

For present-moment treatment, try the following.

- If the pain and throbbing are on the left side of your head, pull your right earlobe upward and outward. Pull as many times as your age (fifty-three times if you're fifty-three years old). Pull as hard as you can tolerate. Ideally, you will hear the crackling "put-put" sound of your earlobe in the beginning. Repeat twice a day for two or three days.
- After pulling your earlobe, fill a basin with warm water and immerse both of your hands in the warm water. Keep adding hot water to maintain the water temperature for thirty minutes.
- When the migraine headache is mild, you'll need only a cold towel on your forehead, covering your eyes. In summertime, use an ice bag. This will cause the blood vessels to constrict, thus relieving the symptoms.
- If the migraine is in both temples, press the roots of both ring fingernails (Jiagung) on both hands. If the migraine affects only one side, apply cutting pressure to the root of the ring fingernail of the affected side with the fingernail of the index finger of the other hand.

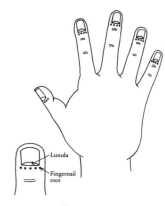

Jiagung

If you find any of these alternatives to drugs can actually prevent attacks, then you will be able to avoid medication. However, many new drug treatments are now available and they offer much hope to the millions who suffer chronic headaches.

Motion Sickness

When we're in a car or on a boat, we are moving and everything around us is moving. This puts our nerves at a disadvantage and disables our equilibrium. Some people's sense of balance is so sensitive that even slight movement can cause sickness. The following two acupressure exercises can steady the central nervous system, control vomiting, and help ease heart palpitations. Additional advice is also offered.

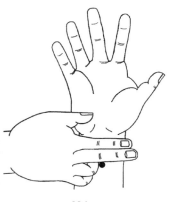

Neiguan

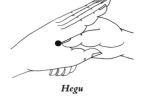

Hegu

- Press the Neiguan point of your right wrist with your left thumb for two minutes (bend your right wrist slightly to feel and locate the exact point). You should feel some pain and numbness. Repeat with your right thumb on the Neiguan point of your left wrist.
- Apply pressure with your left thumb on the Hegu point of your right hand for one to two minutes. You should feel soreness and numbness. Repeat with your right thumb on the Hegu point of your left hand. *Note:* If you are pregnant, or think you might be pregnant, don't do this exercise.
- Try to sit in the front seat or in the center when traveling in a car or boat. Look as far ahead as you can and fix your sight on a point that is not moving. Do not move your eyesight with the motion of the car or ship. In addition, try to eat a light meal before boarding a vehicle or ship, and wear a belt tightly cinched around your waist.

Muscle Spasm of the Chest Wall

What we are addressing here is pain in the chest wall caused by trauma to the chest cavity and its surrounding muscles. The affected muscles go into spasm— they become hyperactive, causing extreme and sudden contractions of the muscles, making breathing difficult and painful. Used in a timely manner, the following exercises help you to breathe normally.

- Breathe in deeply and then hold your breath. Hit forcefully with your fists on both sides of your chest cavity starting from the upper chest and moving downward. Then exhale slowly. Repeat this several times. This process will relax the wall of your breathing muscles as well as reduce the pain in the chest.

• Lie on your back on the floor or a hard bed and turn from side to side. Breathe deeply while turning. This is another method to relieve pain.

Muscle Pain

Pain can occur in any muscle of the body, but it usually occurs in overused muscles. Poor muscle tone may also be the cause, especially when muscles are used extensively. There are ways to prevent muscle pain. Avoid foods that tend to cause muscles to contract. Stay away from peanuts, bananas, fried food, and delicacies such as sea cucumber and seaweed that are commonly found in Japanese, Chinese, and other Asian cuisine.

If you have an acute attack, it's best to have a doctor's treatment and approval before trying the following exercises.

• Rub, press, massage, and pat the affected area for approximately five minutes, two to three times daily. Keep the affected area warm. Should pain recur, massage the area surrounding the affected muscle slowly and deliberately. Concentrate your massage on the area or point that is most sensitive and painful to the touch.

• If the first exercise does not work and pain persists, try the deep-breathing method. Exhale everything that's in the abdomen. Then inhale slowly and deliberately to fill yourself with air. Then slowly and deliberately exhale. This is a way to relax your nerves and muscles, thereby eliminating pain.

Myopia

Most people with myopia, or nearsightedness, need to wear prescription glasses to see well. If you have mild myopia, these exercises can help.

• Massage the main myopic point with your thumb. This point is below the Tsuanzhu point, on the rim of your eye socket. You

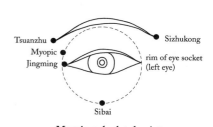

Myopic and related points

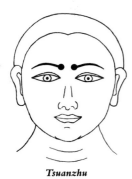

Tsuanzhu

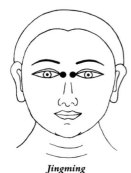

Jingming

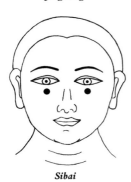

Sibai

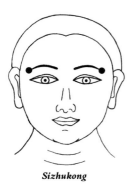

Sizhukong

should feel a slight depression in the bone structure of the eye and experience mild pain, numbness, and heat while applying pressure. When you have located the point, lightly rotate your thumb at that place for twenty minutes.

- With both index fingers, rub the Tsuanzhu, the Jingming, the Sibai, and the Sizhukong points on both sides for two minutes. Do this twice daily. After performing the exercise, close your eyes and rest awhile.

- Take care of your eyes: read while sitting up, not lying down. Do not read in a moving vehicle. Use proper lighting for reading and writing. Watch television moderately. If you are a frequent computer user, shield your monitor with a screen.

- To prevent myopia and preserve good eyesight, do the following exercises.

  After prolonged reading and writing, open and close your eyes slowly. When you close your eyes, close tightly. Slow blinks give a light massage that relaxes your eyes and lubricates your eyeballs.

  Rub your hands to generate heat, then close your eyes lightly. Cover your eyes with your palms on the cheekbones and fingers on the forehead for about a minute.

  Stand approximately four to five feet away from a window. Look at the four corners of the window one at a time, starting with the upper left corner and proceeding clockwise. After staring at each corner, blink your eyes several times. Repeat this exercise five times, then close your eyes for a brief rest. Do the same exercise again, this time moving counterclockwise five times. You will improve your eyesight after prolonged and regular practice of this exercise.

  After reading, writing, or working on a project for an hour or two, rest five to ten minutes before resuming work. Try to look out the window, ideally at a view of mountains and trees. Also look as far away as you can at whatever you can see (preferably at mountains and trees) to help your eyes adapt to looking at objects at various distances.

Neck and Shoulder Pain

Neck and shoulder pain can be caused by a sudden jolt of the neck muscle, exposure to a cold draft while sleeping, prolonged desk work without breaks, and overuse or improper use of a group of muscles. Try the following exercise to get relief.

- In order to treat neck or shoulder pain, apply heavy pressure to the area 2–4 cun directly above the elbow crease in line with your thumb on the affected side. Use the second and middle fingers of the other hand. You should distinctly feel soreness and pain while applying pressure.

    While pressing on these points, keep moving the neck or shoulder until you feel relief. Do the exercise at least three times a day to gain the desired result.

Nosebleeds

When the tiny blood vessels in the nose rupture, blood streams down from your nostrils. The following techniques will help to stop nosebleeds caused by trauma, dryness, localized inflammation, or by minor injury to the lining of the nasal passages. If you begin to experience cold sweats and dizziness, see a doctor without delay.

- When your nose is bleeding, pinch the hollow behind the anklebone. If the source of the blood is from the left nostril, pinch the right foot, and vice versa. If you are pregnant, or think you might be pregnant, skip this exercise.
- If blood is coming from the left nostril, raise the right hand, and if blood is coming from the right nostril, raise the left hand. If both are bleeding, raise both hands. Stand erect when you raise your hands directly over your head.
- Press the antihelix on the ear (the prominent semicircular ridge) with the middle fingers of both hands to close the ear canals for two minutes. The force of your pressure should be strong but tolerable.

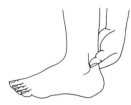

Nosebleed point

- A cold towel or ice pack applied on the nose is also helpful. Sit back and lean slightly forward. Do not blow your nose after the bleeding has stopped.

Numbness of the Hands and Fingers

We all know that sudden weakness or numbness of hands and fingers may be warning signs of stroke and that we need to call an ambulance and get to a hospital in a timely manner to minimize brain injury. You can try these exercises if you have been treated for high blood pressure and stroke and are still having frequent numbness of your hands and fingers. If the numbness of fingers and hands is due to excessive work with fingers—writing, knitting, and so on— these exercises will also help.

- Stretch all ten fingers and put both hands together, placing them in front of your chest. Rub them vigorously for three minutes.
- Whenever possible, rub the tip of the second finger with the thumb and second fingers of the other hand. Alternately rub the other second finger.

Obesity

Excess weight can be hazardous to your health by increasing the risk of diseases such as diabetes, hypertension, atherosclerosis, heart disease, gout, and gallstones.

Although medical conditions can be the cause of obesity, most people gain weight because they eat more than their bodies need. To lose weight you must expend more energy than your total food intake, change your eating habits, and exercise. There are many books on exercise and diet available. Choose a healthy diet that includes plenty of vegetables, fruits, and wheat products. Stay away from sugar, sweets, oils, and fat, and limit salt intake. Drink plenty of juice and water. If you are a fast eater, learn to chew more and chew more slowly. A good basic principle for staying healthy is to make dinner the lightest meal of the day. Eat no food prior going to bed in the evening.

The following suggestions will help you lose weight.

- Try to incorporate physical exercise such as jogging or long walks into your routine to help keep your muscles firm and assist in weight loss. Step climbing is by far the simplest and safest. You will not only see your weight go down, but stabilize as well.

   Walk up and down three flights of stairs nine to ten times each day. If you do this on six flights of stairs, then four to five times each day will suffice. Increase both the frequency and speed gradually. If you do this exercise persistently for at least six months, the result is almost guaranteed. This simple exercise is not only effective in reducing weight and tightening the muscles, but also is a way to give the heart a good workout. Always hold on to railings when going up or down the stairs as a safety precaution.

- Any kind of moving around will keep pounds from stacking up.

Overexertion of the Leg Muscles and Feet

After a vigorous workout such as long-distance walking or cycling, your legs may suddenly feel sharp muscle pain. This is generally due to impaired blood flow to leg muscles, increased metabolic waste, or hypoxia (a defeciency of oxygen reaching the body tissues).

For people with arthritis, muscle pain can also be caused by weather changes. Cold weather can cause the flow of blood and lymphatic fluid to slow down. If you are unable to move your legs even when resting, you need to get medical help to rule out a fracture or a dislocation.

Here are two exercises to alleviate cramps.

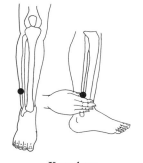

Xuanzhong

Step 1. Massage the following points in this sequence: the Xuanzhong point, the Chengshan point, and then the Yanglingchuan point with your thumb and second finger. Massage each point for one to two minutes.

Step 2. Push with your palms from where the pain and soreness emanate in an upward direction for ten minutes.

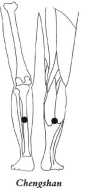

Chengshan   *Yanglingchuan*

Step 1. Sit on a chair and place the right foot on the left thigh. Make a fist with the left hand and apply a moderate amount of petrolium jelly or cold cream to the back of the hand and finger joints. Thoroughly massage the toes, the sole, and the heel of the right foot with the fist for one to two minutes.

Step 2. Vigorously rub the back of the right foot with both thumbs. Starting from the toes, move toward the ankle, then work from the ankle back to the toes. Do this two times.

Step 3. Hold a toe of the right foot with your hand. Pull lightly while rotating the toe. Do this to each toe for one to two minutes.

Step 4. Hold the right foot with both hands. Move the right foot up, down, and sideways to relax the ankle joint for one to two minutes.

Repeat this exercise with the left foot.

To prevent overexertion of the leg muscles and feet, do the following.

Step 1. Stretch your leg forward, move your foot up, down, and sideways.

Step 2. Stretch your toes out for a few seconds, then curl up the toes for a few more seconds.

Step 3. Stand on your toes for a few minutes, then stand on your feet for a few minutes.

Step 4. Stand facing a wall. With one arm on the wall, lean your body toward the wall with both feet firmly planted on the floor. Count slowly to ten.

If you are a runner or cyclist and your feet tire easily, do steps 1 through 3 ten times daily, and step 4 once daily, with your shoes off.

Painful Heels

Painful heels are more prevalent in middle-aged women, especially when they are overweight, because: Some have too little cushioning tissue between the bones and skin of their feet. As the bones start to degenerate due to aging, the heels become very tender. At times the arch collapses as a result of osteoporosis, and the pressure point moves toward the heels. Chronic infection or excessive use of the feet may also cause painful heels. Or a person may have sustained an injury to the foot or have a deformity.

Here are some self-help treatments.

- When the pain is acute, bed rest or taking the weight off the feet is recommended. Placing soft cushions in your shoes may also alleviate the pain somewhat.
- Roll your heels with a rolling pin or a bottle twice daily, thirty minutes each time. Immerse your feet in warm water each night to increase blood circulation to the feet. Continue this exercise for at least seven days. If this does not work, surgery may be required.

Preventing Cancer

Several years back, a professor in Japan stated in his published paper on preventing cancer that he rubbed his patients' backs with towels. His theory was that in our subcutaneous system there lies a certain immune cell. These cells are dormant in normal situations. When your back is rubbed, the rubbing creates heat that hastens the blood flow. At the same time, rubbing stimulates the normally dormant cells. Upon activation, these cells search out, organize an attack on, and break down or gobble up any cells that are foreign, dangerous, or cancerous. In other words, the immune system is boosted and cancer is prevented.

Doctor Wu Song-shein, the noted physician during the Chin dynasty (seventeenth century), frequently stated that back rubs or gua sa can be useful in treating most intestinal ailments. The aborigines and peasants in parts of China still use the back of a large comb made of animal horn as a major medical tool. With the comb dipped in ointment, cold cream, or water, they scrape patients' backs thoroughly to treat the flu or common cold as well as various other ailments such as vomiting, diarrhea, and heatstroke. Refer to chapter 9 for more detail on this massage technique.

The An-Hua Medical School Hospital of China conducted an experiment on patients. They treated patients using the thumb-pushing method of back massage for ten minutes. Blood tests before and after the massage revealed that the amount of total white blood cells increased an average of 19.7 percent. The potency of white blood cells that fight bacteria increased by 34.4 percent.

Since 1984, Dr. Yen has been showing patients with early-stage cancer as well as patients who have had surgery the proper way to rub their backs regularly. Most patients who use back rubs feel better, eat better, sleep better, and are less prone to catch colds. The potential benefit of increasing the immune system with no possible side effects is another reason that the back rub is a good method of cancer prevention.

The reason that traditional Chinese medicine considers back rubs essential is that acupressure points connected to some of the major organs are distributed on both sides of the back. Regularly massaging the back ensures smooth energy flow to the major organs.

- With both hands holding opposite ends of a back scrubber or a dry bath towel, thoroughly rub your back from top to bottom and side to side for ten minutes or more. Do this daily. You can start with two to three minutes and increase gradually to ten. When your skin is red and feels hot, you've reached the desired condition. Protect your back from drafts because this will diminish the effect of the rub. If you feel too weak or have just recovered from an illness or operation, find someone to rub your back for you.

- Exercise such as jogging may also lower the risk of cancer directly and indirectly.

  While exercising, your breathing rate and depth tend to increase. Similar to modern respiratory therapy, excercise increases your pulmonary function.

  Exercise generates perspiration. Some of the oxidants that cause cancer are more readily discharged as a result of perspiring.

  Exercise can enhance the production of white blood cells that fight cancer cells.

  Exercise can increase your blood circulation. Cancer cells are like little grains of sand in a bubbling stream—they can't stand still or expand when blood flow increases.

  Several clinical studies suggest that some cancer patients suffered emotionally before the onset of the disease. Exercise can improve your mood.

  Exercise can improve your physical stamina and build the confidence and persistence necessary to fight cancer.

- Today it is common knowledge that lifestyle is closely related to cancer risk. Most recently, a report published by a major public health institute states that nearly 70 percent of all cancer can be attributed to smoking, eating, and drinking habits, or a sedentary lifestyle. The report further suggests that we should avoid prolonged exposure to the sun's ultraviolet rays, which cause more than 90 percent of skin cancers.

Quitting Smoking

According to a report published by the World Health Organization, every year at least one million people die prematurely as a result of smoking. In 1996, 140,000 new lung cancer cases were diagnosed in the United States alone. Nearly 90 percent of lung cancer patients and one-third of all other cancer patients are smokers. The latest research finds that smokers who quit smoking—even temporarily—heal faster from wounds and surgery. After a person smokes a cigarette, the nerves that constrict blood vessels take twenty minutes to return to normal.

If you have wanted to stop smoking but haven't been able to, here are some ways to help you quit and alleviate your craving for tobacco.

- Forcefully pinch the Liechue and Yangxi points with the thumb and index fingernail of the other hand. Apply the pressure vertically. You should feel a distinct soreness. Practice this on both hands for at least twenty minutes each time, twice daily, over a period of four days. At the end of the first four days, you should have less desire to reach for a cigarette. At the end of eight days (after a second series) you should have no desire for a cigarette. In fact, you'll feel nauseated when someone around you smokes. The success rate using this method is 70 percent.

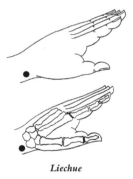

Liechue

- Use mind control.

    In the first several weeks of quitting smoking, stay away from people who smoke or from places where smoking is permitted.

    If you really crave a cigarette, try the delaying tactic by stalling for several minutes. If this doesn't work, try visualization. Imagine the smoke filling your lungs. Or see your health improving after you quit smoking—you can breathe more

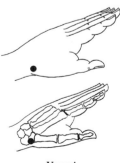

Yangxi

easily and you're full of energy as a result. Ask yourself: "What would happen to me if I continued to smoke?"

Instead of reaching for a cigarette, breathe deeply, jog slowly, join a health club, or pick up a new hobby such as gardening. Chew food or vegetables that are low in calories, such as celery and carrots, since most people tend to gain weight while trying to quit smoking.

Rheumatoid Arthritis

Rheumatoid arthritis begins as an inflammation in the synovial membrane. The synovial membrane produces the fluid that lubricates the joints. When the synovial membrane becomes inflamed, the blood supply to the membrane increases; white blood cells gather in the membrane, and swelling occurs. The swelling can become severe enough to cause deformity of the joint. The inflammation causes the synovial membrane to release chemicals called lysosomal enzymes that destroy cartilage and bone. The body tries to repair the damage but usually forms irregular patches and rough bumps. These outgrowths aggravate the problem and decrease joint function.

The cause of the inflammation is still unclear. Many medical researchers theorize that the body's immune system mistakenly attacks the joints. Diet and stress are often mentioned as being responsible for initiating the inflammation. The most remarkable clinical symptoms are the symmetrical and multiple locations of the inflammation, predominantly in the hand, wrist, and toe joints. In the earlier stage the symptoms are redness, swelling, pain, and difficulty in movement. As the disease progresses, the joints become stiff, hard, and deformed. Some patients also exhibit symptoms such as fever, lethargy, and weight loss. The disease could take years to run its course. The seriousness of the disease can increase and decrease intermittently.

To date, there is no known effective cure, nor are there ways to reverse the preexisting damage. The medical world and major pharmaceutical concerns are racing to find ways to halt the development and worsening of the disease. These self-massage exercises are a means to that end.

- In order to control the disease from progressing and to revive function in the area, utilize all possible available time to massage, kneed, rub, and push the area several times daily. With the help of another person, passively bend, stretch, and turn the joint as often as possible. You should feel some relief after the massage. At least three times a day, submerge your body in hot water for approximately ten minutes. Keep the water temperature constant by adding hot water to the tub while soaking. This is better than taking painkillers, if time permits.

- Keeping yourself reasonably active is important to keeping the joints from becoming deformed. When the disease is active, you need to give the afflicted joints sufficient rest. However, some joint movement is helpful to improve mobility. For example, you can do some bending and stretching while lying on the floor or in bed. The purpose is to enhance the power of the surrounding muscle and to prevent the joint from being deformed. If you just lie in bed and give your afflicted joints plenty of rest, you may inadvertently cause the muscles to atrophy and speed up the progress of the disease. If you suffer poor appetite, eat food high in protein, minerals, and vitamins. Eat a balanced diet. Stay away from high-calorie food if you are overweight.

Ringing in the Ears (Tinnitus)

Ringing in the ears can be attributed to working in severely high temperatures, constipation, cold, headache, and toothache. High blood pressure, high cholesterol, and heavy smoking affect your ears before they affect your heart. Therefore, ringing in the ears may be an early warning sign of an eventual heart attack. If you have high blood pressure or high blood cholesterol and are over fifty, and the ringing in the ears persists or worsens, have your heart function checked out as soon as possible.

If you can hear a ringing or buzzing sound that is occasionally loud and at times faint and which interferes with your normal hearing, try these two self-help exercises. They will not alleviate a ringing sound caused by a heavy blast, food poisoning, or diseases of the ear canal—you'll need to consult a physician for help with those problems.

- Press the root of the left index fingernail, ring fingernail, and little

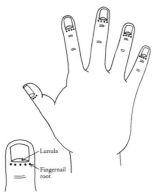

Jiagung

fingernail (Jiagung) with the tip of your right thumb or index finger for three to five minutes each. Do the same with your left thumb or index finger on your right hand.

- Cover your ear canals with the palms of both hands. Gently tap the back of your head with your fingers while opening and closing the canals with a steady rhythm. Do this exercise once in the morning and once in the evening for five to six minutes each time.

In addition to using these methods, you'll also need to get adequate rest and exercise and avoid emotional outbursts and sexual intercourse.

Shingles

Shingles is a very painful disease that more often occurs in women than men, in older people than young, and on one side of the body than both. It is a viral infection of the underlying tissues and nerves. It can be triggered by fatigue, poor health, cancer, sudden onset of cold weather, and various other diseases.

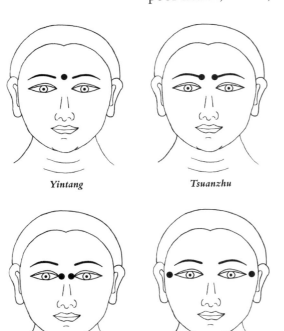

Yintang

Tsuanzhu

Jingming

Taiyan

Patients have described the pain as that of many prickling needles, knife stabs, or electrical shock.

A nutritious diet, adequate rest, and control of stress—all essential to a healthy immune system—can help in recovering from shingles, and possibly in preventing it. Early treatment is the key. As soon as there is an unexplained rash or pain in any part of the body, contact your physician for treatment and prescriptions of painkillers and antiviral agents. He may also provide treatment to protect the eyes.

Try the following massages as well.

- While sitting or lying down with eyes closed, press and rub all sides of the bone structure of the affected eye area with your thumb and index finger. The pressure should be as much as you can tolerate for four to five minutes.
- Follow by pressing these points for one minute

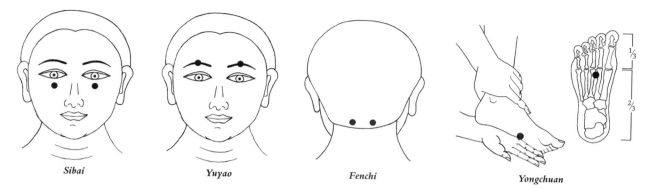

Sibai   Yuyao   Fenchi   Yongchuan

each: Yingtang, Tsuanzhu, Jingming, Taiyan, Sibai, and Yuyao points of the affected side, and Fenchi points on both sides.

- Rub the Yongchuan points of both feet with your palms for two minutes each.

Shortness of Breath

Shortness of breath and having a winded or bottled-up feeling in the chest are more prevalent among people who do desk work for long hours or who work in an environment of high room temperature with poor ventilation. Exhaustion, heatstroke, cold, nervousness, insomnia, and dehydration can all cause a stuffy sensation in the chest and shortness of breath.

These are exercises you can do for relief. Pick one that you are comfortable with.

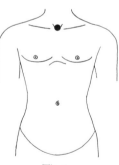

Tiantu

- Lie down on your back, push gently with the palms of both hands from the Tiantu point toward the Danzhong point. Repeat at least four times.
- With the surfaces of both thumbs, rub from the tips of your collarbones downward to the Danzhong point. Then press and massage each rib from top to bottom, moving from the center outward. This exercise will also mitigate any pain in the rib area.
- Insert the tip of your middle finger into your Tiantu point. Try to go deeper into the Tiantu point, which is hollow, while inhaling. Let go quickly while exhaling.
- Place your left hand on the tip of the collarbone. Then make a fist with your right hand and hit or tap your left hand three times forcefully. You

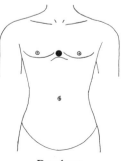

Danzhong

should feel relief afterward. *Note:* This is not recommended if you have a heart condition.

- Another effective remedy is to press the roots of your left middle and little fingernails (Jiagung) with the tip of your right thumb or index fingernail for three to five minutes. Repeat on the right hand.

Sinusitis

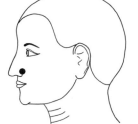

Bizuan

Sinusitis is the inflammation of the membranes lining the air spaces in the skull. It is often accompanied by headaches, dull pain, runny nose, and tenderness around the eyes or cheekbones.

If you suffer from recurrent sinusitis, try the following massages.

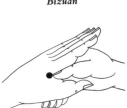

Hegu

- There are four pressure points that you should massage alternately in two groups. The first group is made up of the Bizuan (nostril) and the Hegu points, with Bizuan being the main point and Hegu the supplementary point. Apply a cutting pressure to the left Bizuan point with your right thumb. Then do the same to the left Hegu point with your right thumb. Reverse the process on the right side. *Note:* If you are pregnant, or think you might be pregnant, skip the Hegu point.
- The second group is made up of the Yingxiang and Shaosheng points, the Yingxiang being the main point and the Shaosheng the supplementary point. First apply cutting pressure to the right Yingxiang point and the right Shaosheng points with your left thumb. Do the same on the left side.

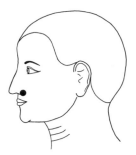

Yingxiang

Massage both groups twice daily for ten minutes each. Spend three minutes at a time on the main points and two minutes on the supplementary points.

Stiff Neck

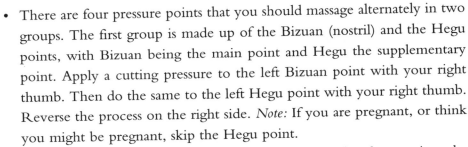

Shaosheng

If you sleep with many pillows, or with hard pillows, or in a drafty area, you may wake up to find that you cannot move your neck and that your neck is stiff, sore, and painful on one side. If the pain is in the middle of the back of the neck and accompanied by numbness of your arm or fingers, it may be associated with the spine. If this is the case you will need to consult a doctor for proper diagnosis and treatment.

Try these exercises for a stiff neck.

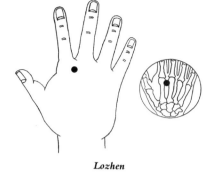

Lozhen

- Rub the tip of the middle finger of the affected side with your thumb and index finger of the other hand. Rub gradually toward the base of the middle finger and move your head and neck slowly for three minutes. Then lightly tap the affected area with your fist for one minute.
- Apply pressure on the Lozhen point on the back of the hand of the affected side with the thumb of your opposite hand. When rubbing and pressing this point, you should feel a distinct soreness and numbness. At the same time, bend your head so that your chin touches your chest, and then raise it. Then turn your head to the left three times and to the right three times. If the pain extends to both sides of the neck, apply pressure on the Lozhen points of both hands.
- Stand or sit straight, then drop your head and chin into the neck as far as possible. Raise both shoulders so that your earlobes almost touch your shoulders. Then stick your neck out and drop your shoulders in a sudden motion. Repeat this exercise twenty times.

In a more severe case, lie down and rest after the exercise. Apply a heating pad or wrap your neck in a dry towel.

Stomach Pain

The classic symptom of a duodenal ulcer is pain in the upper abdomen. The pain feels like gnawing, burning, or cramping, and usually occurs within one to three hours after a meal. Belching, bloating, or intolerance of fatty foods are also common symptoms. Other than the self-help measures outlined here, adequate rest, proper diet, and lifestyle changes are key ingredients for a speedy recovery.

- Peck like a bird. When you sense that you are about to have a heartburn attack, lie down and relax your stomach muscles. Place your palm on your

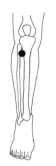

Zusanli

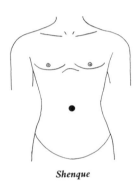

Shenque

stomach. Tap your stomach with your fingers slightly bent, like a bird pecking (hence the name), three to four times per second. The up and down pecking motion should be even and gentle. Start from the upper part of your stomach and gradually move to your navel. Going back and forth, alternate with both hands for ten minutes. You should be able to hear your stomach moving. If you can pass gas, relief should ensue. This massage can also help if you feel bloated or have abdominal cramps.

- Massage your legs. Press the Zusanli points of both legs with either your thumbs or middle fingers for three to five minutes. You should feel soreness and numbness and then relief.

- To prevent heartburn, do the following massage exercises daily.

  Ring around the abdomen. Lie on your back and relax your abdominal muscles. Using the navel, or Shenque point, as the center of the circle, massage clockwise with your palm one hundred times. Then alternate with the other hand, massaging counterclockwise one hundred times. The massage pressure should be strong yet gentle. This will improve your digestive system enormously.

  Press your navel (Shenque point). Sit or lie down and slowly press your navel with your thumb. Push slowly but forcefully from your navel downward and gradually release. Do this twenty times. This massage also relieves constipation.

  The ideal time for either exercise is once in the morning and once at bedtime.

Note: All the exercises and massages are preventive. If you have black stools or severe stomach pain, don't do the exercises. Consult your doctor for possible gastrointestinal bleeding. You should also consult your doctor without delay if you're vomiting, have unexplained weight loss, difficulty swallowing, or persistent or worsening pain.

Stress—Mental and Physical Fatigue

Illness can cause fatigue. Strenuous physical labor can cause physical fatigue. Mental fatigue is yet another type of fatigue.

Mental fatigue manifests itself in various forms. In some instances, after you have immersed yourself in extensive paperwork, meetings, and stressful situations, you may feel nauseated, forgetful, and unable to concentrate. Sometimes prolonged work or working the night shift may also cause headaches, tiredness, diminished attention span, and indigestion. Long meetings and heated discussions can also induce mental fatigue. (You cannot alleviate depression with massage.)

Most people who suffer either physical or mental stress yawn often. They support their chins with both hands or put their feet up on the table. Recent research suggests that mental stress can cause insufficient blood flow to the heart, putting those people at high risk of having a heart attack. They tend to use alcohol, cigarettes, caffeine, and spicy food to keep themselves alert and interested. If you fit this description, try these methods of alleviating stress instead.

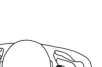

Yongchuan

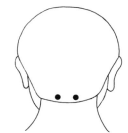

Laogong

- To relieve mental stress, apply heavy pressure on these points in the following sequence.

    The Yongchuan points on the soles of your feet. This is a major point that controls the ch'i and blood circulation in your body.

    The Laogong points in the centers of your palms.

    The Jianjing points on both shoulders, midway between the seventh cervical vertebra, and the tip of the clavicle.

    The Fenchi points in the back of your neck. The Fenchi points can help to eliminate the pressure built up within you.

Jianjing

Fenchi

- Another way to relieve stress is to close your eyes and press your ears with both palms. While tapping the back of your head with your index fingers, tap your upper teeth with your lower teeth. Repeat ten times. Bring both palms away from your ears for a few seconds, then repeat the exercise several times. You should feel relief, especially if you feel light-headed or faint.
- Aside from massages, if you have overworked either physically, mentally, or both, take time to exercise and maintain a balanced lifestyle.

Sty

A sty is a boil-like infection, often at the base of the eyelash. It's caused by inflammation of one or more of the sebaceous glands of the eyelids. Traditional Chinese doctors believe that excessive intake of hot and spicy food irritates the digestive system and a sty is a manifestation of the overheating of that system.

Other than warm soaks, you can can use acupressure massage to mitigate the redness and swelling of the sty. Once the sty bursts and pus begins to come out, stop the massage.

Try these acupressure points.

- Starting from the inner corner of the affected eye at the Taiyan point, rub with the base of your thumb for three minutes. Although some pressure is necessary, be gentle and swift in your movements. The object of this massage is to improve circulation in the surrounding area of the affected eye.
- Follow this by rubbing repeatedly the following points: Jingming, Tsuanzhu, Yuyao, Sizhukong, Tongzilliao, Taiyan, and Sibai. Use your index finger and continue the massage for five minutes.

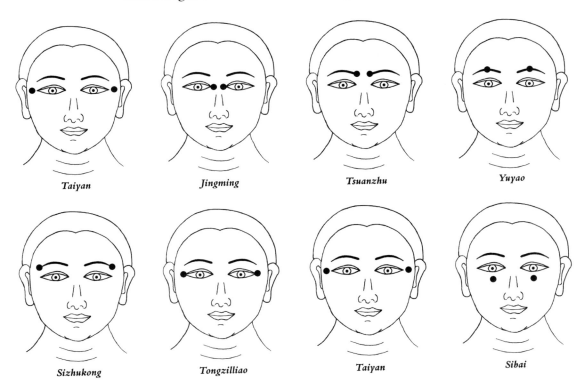

Taiyan   Jingming   Tsuanzhu   Yuyao

Sizhukong   Tongzilliao   Taiyan   Sibai

If none of the above works and the eye becomes red and painful, consult your doctor.

Swollen Legs and Sore Back

Constant leg swelling may be associated with inefficient metabolism. It is the consensus of the traditional Chinese doctors that leg swelling and sore back (pain in one side of your back just above the waist) is related closely to the function or malfunction of the lungs, kidneys, and spleen. Excessive standing or sitting, fatigue, and severely cold temperatures can all result in a sore back and swollen legs.

These exercises can alleviate the problem.

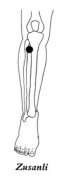

Zusanli

- Massage the left middle finger from the tip to the wrist (in a straight line) with your right thumb and index finger for three minutes. Then do the same to your right middle finger.
- Press the Zusanli and Yanglingchuan points with your fingers for two minutes each, first on the left leg and then on the right leg.

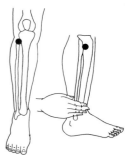

Yanglingchuan

Practice both massages twice daily. Ideally do the evening routine just before you are ready to go to bed. This will not only make your leg swelling diminish or disappear but will also improve your stomach and intestinal functions.

If your leg swelling and soreness in the waist are accompanied by tiredness, diarrhea, and intermittent fever and cold chills, see your doctor without delay.

Tonsillitis and Throat Infection

Acute tonsillitis and throat infection are generally considered infections of the upper respiratory system. These two can appear together or separately. If you are overworked and your body is at a low point of resistance, bacteria and viruses are prone to invade your body through your throat and tonsils.

The onset of both acute tonsillitis and throat infection is often sudden. One day you are fine and the next day you have chills and fever. Complaints such as body aches, headaches, throat pain, earaches, and difficulty swallowing are

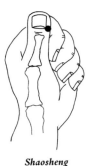

Shaosheng

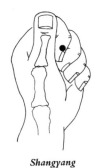

Shangyang

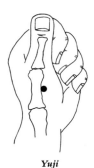

Yuji

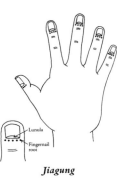

Lunula
Fingernail root

Jiagung

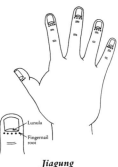

Hegu

common. If you see redness and swelling on both sides of the throat, at times with whitish or yellowish spots, and the lymph nodes behind your jaws are swollen and painful to the touch, chances are you have acute tonsillitis or a throat infection. It is best to consult a physician immediately.

Try the following massages as preventive measures.

- Apply cutting pressure to the Shaosheng and Shangyang points on your left hand with the tip of your right thumb. First apply the pressure parallel to the point and then perpendicularly. Do the same with your right hand.

- If your throat hurts, pinch the Hegu points on both hands. Pinch as hard as you can tolerate. Repeat the massage two or three times daily. The Hegu point is an essential pain-relieving point for toothache, headache, and stomachache. This point is also effective in lowering fever and treating infections. *If you're pregnant or suspect that you may be pregnant, stay away from this point.*

- Apply cutting pressure to the root points of the thumbs, index fingernails, and ring fingernails (Jiagung) on both hands with the tip of your thumb or index fingernail for five minutes at each point.

- Apply cutting pressure to the Yuji points on both hands with your thumb and second finger. You will feel soreness. Then try swallowing repeatedly to relieve the pain in your throat. To prevent the throat pain from recurring, also apply cutting pressure to the Hegu point (see above) of both hands for thirty seconds each.

Toothaches

Tooth decay and periodontal disease cause toothaches. You should see a dentist to take care of the problem as soon as practical.

To alleviate the pain, try these self-help methods on a temporary basis.

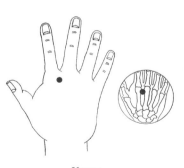

Yatong

- Rub the Yatong (Toothache) point with the thumb and index finger. You should feel some soreness and numbness. Increase the pressure gradually for one to two minutes and your tooth pain should disappear.
- Massage the Hegu point with an ice cube for one to two minutes.
- Apply cutting pressure to the Shangyang point and the Hegu point on your affected side. Do both sides if it is your front tooth. In addition, apply cutting pressure to the Xiaguan point if it is your upper tooth and the Jiache point for the lower tooth. Hold the pressure for one minute on each pressure point.

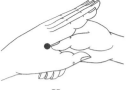

Hegu

- The "reaction points" on the palms are very useful for treating toothaches. To locate the correct reaction point, take the midpoint of the crease at the end of the thumb and the midpoint of the crease at the start of your wrist and draw a straight line linking the two points. The upper half of the line corresponds to the left side of your mouth and the lower half to the right, the left side of the

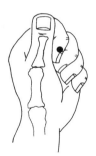

Shangyang

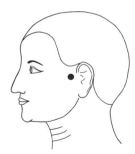

Xiaguan

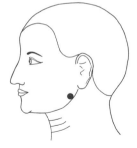

Jiache

line to the upper teeth and the right side of the line to the lower teeth. Depending on the location of your toothache, look at the corresponding quadrant for an area that is either pink or light purple in color. This is the reaction point. Press on the reaction point with a bundle of toothpicks or matchsticks for a minute or more to stop the pain.

Varicose Veins

Varicose veins, or swollen leg veins, are more prevalent in people with jobs that require prolonged standing. Women sometimes develop varicose veins during pregnancy because of pressure on the pelvic veins and inferior vena cava from the baby's weight. When the leg veins are swollen they cause poor circulation in the legs. Varicose veins are most commonly found in the back of the calf and along the inside of the leg.

After prolonged standing, your legs will feel heavy and painful and your ankles will be swollen. Other than the swollen veins, there is little or no pain in the early stage. As the problem progresses, the affected veins will develop a deep color. The poor blood circulation can deprive the affected area of nutrients. A bug bite or an injury can take a long time to heal. Once you have developed varicose veins, you need to treat them aggressively.

- In less severe cases or when surgery is not feasible, you should walk briskly four times daily, fifteen minutes at at time. Fast walking exercises the leg muscles and helps blood to flow upward toward the heart.
- Sit with your legs elevated whenever you can. Wear support stockings or specially prescribed hose. Swimming, walking on bare feet, or flexing your calf muscles can all increase the blood circulation in your legs and improve the health of the leg veins.

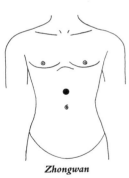

Zhongwan

Vomiting

Vomiting is a physical reaction, usually an indication of an underlying disease of the digestive system. If you have ingested food that has gone bad, it's desirable to expel the poisonous substance by inducing vomiting. However, if you vomit repeatedly, the excessive loss of water and electrolytes can be life threatening. Drink plenty of clear (nonalcoholic) fluids in small sips even if you cannot keep anything down.

Consult your physician as soon as practical. Try the following to temporarily stop the vomiting.

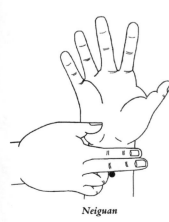

Neiguan

- Press the Zhongwan point with your middle finger for two to three minutes. The Zhongwan point is located approximately 4 cun directly above your navel.
- Press the Neiguan point of your right wrist with your left thumb for two minutes. Bend your right wrist slightly to feel and locate the exact point.

You should feel some pain and numbness. Repeat with your right thumb on the left wrist, two minutes for each.

• Try the gua sa method described in chapter 9.

Younger-Looking Face

Wrinkles and fine lines can be mitigated and minimized if you take care of your health and skin, avoid extensive sun exposure, and massage your face on a regular basis. The direction of the massage should follow the muscle and the blood flow, otherwise your effort is counterproductive. Massage each area ten to fifteen times daily.

• Massage the forehead with your index fingers, starting where the eyebrows meet, in an outward and upward motion.
• Massage the nose with your index fingers, starting where the eyebrows meet, in a downward motion.
• Massage the upper eyelids, starting from the inner corners of the eyes and moving toward the outer corner of the eye. For the lower eyelid, start from the outer corner of the eyes and move inward.
• Massage the upper lip, starting at the middle and moving outward. Do the same for the lower lip.
• Use your fingers to move the neck upward and outward.
• Massage the cheeks upward, starting from the bottom of your face.
• Try washing your face in the same direction as you massage. Use lukewarm water. Persistent use of hot water tends to overrelax your complexion and creates fine wrinkles, whereas extremely cold water will make your complexion dry and flaky. Eat and drink plenty of nutritious food and juice and exercise on a regular basis. Do not massage if you have any wounds, infections, or acne on your face.

5 For Men Only

Early Ejaculation

If you experience early ejaculation during sexual intercourse or ejaculation while sleeping, try the following exercises.

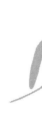

- Rub the Yongchuan point of your left foot with your right palm. Rub until the bottom of your foot feels hot to the touch. Repeat the same on your right foot with your left palm.
- With the backs of both fists, start at the sides of the spine and press downward to the tailbone and then upward as far as your arms can reach. Repeat eighty-one times. The movements should be swift and forceful so that your waist feels the warmth. While doing this exercise, try to exercise your sphincter muscle by holding and releasing it.
- Rub your palms together to create heat and then place your hands on your navel, one on top of the other. Press and rotate your hands clockwise and counterclockwise for one minute each. Then rub between the navel and the area of the pubis one inch below the navel for one minute, alternating hands.

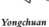

Yongchuan

These exercises should be done once in the morning and once in the evening. Generally, you should notice results from the exercise after ten or more days.

- You should sleep on your left side with no pressure on your heart. Bend your right leg and stretch out your left leg. This is an ideal position for avoiding nightmares and ejaculation while sleeping.

Erection Difficulties

There are many possible sources of erection difficulties. Emotional factors and stress are common causes of impotence. Traditional Chinese medicine relates the sexual function closely with the kidneys. Take a look at your lifestyle and diet and remove any factors that may be overtaxing the kidneys' function. Cut down or stay away from alcohol consumption. If you're taking any medications, particularly antidepressants, antihypertensives, or antianxiety drugs, your failure to have an erection may be a side effect. Discuss it with your physician.

Avoid tight pants that limit the circulation in the genital area. Explore ways to reduce your sexual anxiety by examining the cause of your nervousness and worries. Exercise regularly. If the problem persists, consult your physician to rule out any physiological factors.

The following exercise should help solve erection difficulties.

- Hold your testicles in the palm of your hand. With your other hand, massage in a clockwise direction the middle of the pubis area one inch below the navel. Do this eighty-one times. Change hands and repeat the massage for another eighty-one times, this time counterclockwise. In Taoism, the number of yang, or high positive energy, is nine. Eighty-one represents the highest possible yang energy because it is nine times nine. Do this massage once in the morning and once in the evening.

6 For Women Only

Blocked Milk Duct

Blocked milk duct often occurs to a woman three to four days after childbirth. If you notice a hard, painless lump in your breast or underarm, a blocked milk duct is the most likely cause. Self-massage and continued feeding should clear the lump. If the lump becomes painful or inflamed, see your physician.

Before beginning self-massage, place a hot towel on the affected breast for five minutes. Then try the following massage exercises.

- Place the affected breast in one hand. Apply the four fingers of the other hand (minus the thumb) directly at the base of the affected breast and push the breast in a perpendicular direction toward the center of the breast. Repeat ten to twenty times.
- With the thumb and second fingers, hold the affected breast from the base. Using the other hand as a wedge, start from the area above the breast and push the breast toward the center to clear the milk from the duct.

Alternate both methods repeatedly. The massage should be soft and slow but deliberate. Do not put pressure directly on the lump, but slowly push and squeeze toward it. As the milk moves through, the lump should gradually disappear.

Breast Abscess

Breast abscess or infection in the breast occurs often to women during breast feeding after six months' time. It is at this stage that milk flow is the heaviest. An interruption in breast feeding or an infection could cause a localized breast infection. When you have a blocked milk duct, or an inflamed breast, avoid eating fresh fish and foods that are known to induce more milk. When breasts are swollen, express milk as often as necessary with a breast pump. Keep the baby's mouth clean to protect your nipples from infection.

If you feel feverish and suffer discomfort in the breasts or nipples or all or part of one breast is inflamed, seek the care of a physician as soon as possible. However, before all of one breast is inflamed or within one or two days of discovering a lump, even if you feel a slight fever, self-massage can help.

- This is a self-patting exercise. Either in a standing or sitting position, place the arm of the affected side on a table. Relax the breast and upper body muscle. Pat the affected side with the palm of the healthy side (assuming only one of the breasts is affected). Starting from the middle of the upper arm, pat upward toward the collarbone for thirty minutes. If both breasts are affected, repeat the exercise on the other side. Continue for thirty minutes. Do this exercise again in four to six hours. You should see results in two to three sessions. The main purpose of this exercise is to lightly shake the affected breast and clear the milk duct.
- Here is a folk cure. Dip the back of a comb made of wood or horn in a lanolin ointment or cooking oil. Place the back of the comb on the breast lump and draw the comb toward the nipple. Repeat the massage until milk flows freely again.

Breast Feeding—Before and After Delivery

Breast milk is the ideal food for newborns. It satisfies all the nutritional needs for infants to grow and develop and is the most easily assimilated food for your child. Breast-fed babies develop fewer allergies and are less prone to gastroenteritis. Antibodies in the breast milk provide natural protection for your child against germs. If you plan to breast-feed, begin preparation at the start of the fifth month of pregnancy.

Self-massage is one of the most important elements in the preparation process. At the beginning of the fifth month of pregnancy, milk ducts begin to develop and expand. Massaging the breasts at this time can loosen the structure of the breasts and stimulate blood circulation.

One week after delivery is a critical time to establish successful feeding. Aggressively massage your breasts two to three days after delivery to enable milk to flow freely. Take the following steps to ensure successful breast feeding.

- Prior to delivery, preferably starting around the fifth month of pregnancy, massage your breasts with your hands before going to bed at night. First wash your breasts with a warm wet cloth, then place the warm cloth on the breasts for five minutes. Then massage the sides of your breasts in a clockwise direction. Follow by massaging from the base of the breasts in an upward motion toward the nipples.
- Two to three days after birth, massage before every feeding. The frequency of the massage can increase gradually and should last for ten to fifteen minutes. The sequence is as follows:

  Step 1. Move your fingers around the circumference of the breasts in a clockwise direction. Then raise the breasts with your fingers and pull toward the nipples.

  Step 2. Hold the base of the breasts with both hands. Pull the breasts toward the nipples. Move the breasts up, down, and sideways.

  Step 3. Massage the sides of the breasts by using the opposite hands.

  Step 4. Lift and pull the nipples away from the breasts with the thumbs and second fingers. With a warm cloth wipe away any milk that comes out.

  Step 5. After massaging, express milk from the breasts with the thumbs and second fingers. Usually a light-colored or transparent liquid will ooze out. You are now ready to feed your baby.

Wash your hands prior to massaging your breasts. When massaging one breast, cover the other to keep it warm. Massage lightly in the beginning. Increase the pressure gradually. Never handle yourself roughly.

Difficult Urination after Childbirth

If you experience difficulty in passing urine after childbirth, try one of the following exercises.

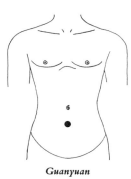

Guanyuan

- Lie on your back. Do ten to twenty sit-ups. This will improve blood circulation and tone the abdominal muscles as well as the pelvic floor muscles that support the bladder and reproductive organs.
- If you have the urge to urinate, but have difficulty getting started, press the Guanyuan point for two minutes or more. The Guanyuan point is located 3 cun below the navel, or Shenque point.
- Press the Linou (Diuretic) point for five to ten minutes, twice daily. The Linou point is located approximately 2.5 cun below the navel, or Shenque point, and 0.5 cun above the Guanyan point. You can use this for any other unstable bladder condition as well.

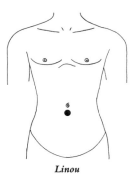

Linou

Fibrous Breasts

A common problem in young and middle-aged women is pain and tenderness in one or both breasts caused by breast lumps. These lumps may be tender and painful to the touch. Symptoms such as fluid retention, nausea, and dry mouth may accompany the lumps. While these symptoms may be a common occurrence—a condition known as fibroadenosis—any lumps in the breast should be examined by a physician to rule out breast cancer.

Once you have determined that the lump is not a malignant tumor, wearing a firm support bra may help reduce the discomfort. Try to rest and stay upbeat in outlook. Avoid eating spicy food. The following exercises may also help.

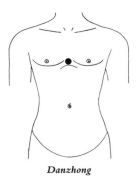

Danzhong

- This massage is known as self-patting. Either sit or lie down. Place the arm of the affected side on a table or bed. Relax the breast and upper muscle. Pat the affected side with the palm of the healthy side (assuming only one of the breasts is affected). Starting from the middle of the upper arm, pat upward to the upper portion of your affected breast for thirty minutes. If both breasts are affected, repeat the same exercise on the other side. Do this exercise every four to six hours. Generally, it takes two to three sessions to achieve satisfactory results.
- Massage from the armpit down to the upper waist of the affected side for two minutes.
- Rub the armpit of the affected side in a circular motion for one to two minutes.
- Rub the Danzhong point in a circular motion for one to two minutes. Apply pressure to the Danzhong point for another half a minute.

Practice these exercises once in the morning and again in the evening. You should feel relief after a few days. It may take six months or longer to be totally well.

Incorrect Position of the Fetus

Whether the fetal position is correct or not will affect the eventual delivery. In most cases of incorrect fetal position, the fetus is situated so that there is a possibility that the buttocks may come through the birth canal before the head.

The following method for encouraging the fetus to turn was developed by a gynecologist in Japan and is simple and easy to follow.

- Lie on a bed on your back with one or two pillows placed under your waist, and hang both legs over the side of the bed. Do this twice daily— once in the morning and again in the evening, each time for fifteen to twenty minutes. This exercise should be practiced over a period of seven days. The position of the fetus will usually correct itself after one or two sessions.

Insufficient Milk Flow

If you have inadequate milk to breast-feed your newborn, you should pay special attention to proper nutrition. Make sure that your diet includes fresh fish, milk, and other foods that will help produce more milk. Get plenty of rest. Also, try this self-massage exercise.

- Place the palm of your hand on the breast; rub and move around repeatedly. Pick up the breast muscle with your fingers and then let go. Do this for ten minutes each time, three to four times daily. This exercise will stimulate the nerves in the breast to send a message to the brain to produce more milk.

Menstrual Discomfort

Menstrual pain often decreases after a woman has had her first child. Some women suffer painful periods throughout the fertile years, however. Severe cramping in the lower abdomen, nausea, and vomiting can occur before or during the period.

If you suffer from menstrual discomfort, try these exercises. However, if you are pregnant (or suspect that you are) do not try these exercises.

- This first exercise is for long-term relief. Lie down and rub your lower abdomen (below the navel) in a clockwise direction for fifteen minutes. Apply pressure to the Guanyuan point for twenty minutes, using alternate hands. Your abdomen should feel sore. Then sit up and rub the Sanyinjiao points on the ankles for two minutes each.

    Start this exercise at least one week prior to your period, practicing it once every evening. Stop when your period ends. If you do this exercise persistently, you should be entirely rid of the menstrual pain after five to seven months.

- This exercise will provide temporary relief. Lie down and rub both hands until they are warm to the touch. Place your warm palms on the lower abdomen directly below the navel. Massage up and down, then left and right. Finally, rub clockwise. Do this with alternating hands, one hand

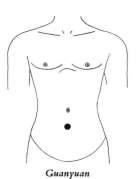

Guanyuan

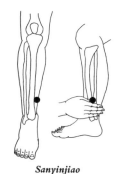

Sanyinjiao

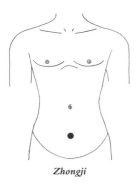

Zhongji

after the other. Stop when you feel warmth in the lower abdomen (in about fifteen minutes). With your thumb, press forcefully the Zhongji point for ten minutes.

- Dropping two to three drops of 70 percent alcohol in both ears should relieve the pain instantly.
- It is the general consensus of most Chinese herbal doctors that young women should take various precautions prior to periods. Avoid strenuous exercise and heavy lifting. Keep your body warm and pay attention to personal hygiene. Eat plenty of vegetables and stay away from food with high sodium content. Sleep and rest adequately to ensure a pain-free period.

Overdue Pregnancy

The average duration of pregnancy is forty weeks. If the pregnancy continues beyond forty-two weeks it may adversely affect the safety of the mother as well as the baby. Your physician may advise you to have the delivery induced. There is a massage that you can do to prevent the pregnancy from extending beyond forty-two weeks.

- Beginning at the thirty-ninth week, apply a warm wet cloth on both breasts. Massage the breasts gently for one hour, three times daily.

Womb Education

According to scientific studies, a six-month-old fetus can hear its mother's heartbeat, voice, and other sounds of the outer world. The fetus also moves in reaction to various sounds. Traditional Chinese doctors have always empha-sized the importance of womb education. They believe that the fetus starts to learn in the mother's womb. Eastern Indians hold a similar belief. In fact, the famous story of Abhimanyu and Shukdev of India is a classic example. It tells how a fetus starts learning within the mother's womb.

The psychological state of a woman during pregnancy directly affects the child's shape and brain development. Self-massage is an effective method of womb education. Try the following technique.

- When you are approximately six months pregnant you should be able to feel the head, body, and extremities of your baby. At that time, you can softly rub or pat the fetus. Prior to going to bed in the evening, lie in a supine position and relax your abdominal muscles. Place both hands on the abdomen and lightly massage the baby in an upward motion for five minutes at a time. Rest for a few minutes and repeat.

During pregnancy, avoid unpleasant stimulation. Try to enjoy artistic objects such as pleasant paintings and flowers. Take a stroll in the garden or visit scenic places as often as you can. Maintain a stable and cheerful mood. In addition, listening to beautiful, soothing music can help both the mother and the child. Pay special attention to proper exercise and proper nutrition.

The expectant father can help in all these activities and contribute by keeping the expectant mother happy during these vital days of pregnancy.

PART THREE

Wellness for Life

7 A Daily
Wellness Program

The Deep-Breathing Method

This breathing technique is a basic exercise of the Buddhist monks. By taking long, deep breaths you will recharge your ch'i and help your body heal itself.

- Stand, sit, or lie down. Lean your upper body slightly forward if you are standing or sitting down. Put one hand on your chest, the other on your abdomen. When you exhale, empty all the air from the abdomen slowly and deliberately. At the same time lightly press the hand down on the abdomen. When you inhale, inhale as much air as you can into your abdomen by allowing your abdomen to extend outward. The rate of exhaling should be two or three times slower than the rate of inhaling. Inhale through your nose and exhale through your mouth in a whistling motion. Breathe seven to eight times per minute.

Practice deep breathing at least once in the morning—facing the sunrise if possible—and once in the evening. Do this exercise for ten to twenty minutes at a time.

Always breathe with a regular rhythm—deeply, gently, and effortlessly. Once you have mastered the breathing technique, your hands will no longer have to be on the chest or abdomen.

A Five-Minute Daily Exercise—Anytime, Anywhere

Nowadays, although more and more people are aware of the importance of taking care of their bodies, finding enough time to exercise is a dominant issue. The following is a simple exercise devised for young and middle-aged readers who are "on the go." It only takes five minutes. Try to do it daily or at least five times a week. Keep this in mind: If you can sit up, do not lie down. If you can stand up, do not sit down. If you can be active do not stand idle.

Step 1. Bend both knees to lower your body as far as you can manage. Do this fifty to sixty times.

Step 2. Stand erect and face a wall. The distance between you and the wall should be at least an arm's length, and preferably more. Stretch your arms and touch the wall with both hands. Bring your upper body close against the wall. Push your body away from the wall with both hands. Repeat this exercise until you feel tired. Increase the duration of the exercise as you build up stamina.

Massage to Stay Healthy—From Middle to Old Age

When Dr. Yen studied with the monk, he stayed in Lin-Yan She, a Buddhist temple in Fuchow, China, for a couple of years. He observed that many monks were seventy years or older but were in remarkably good health. They led a very disciplined life and followed a set timetable of eating and sleeping. They suffered no heart, lung, intestinal, or other significant diseases. None had had any surgeries, major or minor. They had their own hair and teeth. Their minds were keen and lucid. There were no noticeable age spots or wrinkles on their faces. They were agile and their backs were straight. They had only minor ailments, which they took care of themselves with self-treatment or herbal medicines. When asked about their secret formula, they attributed their long and healthy lives to practicing self-massage and inner exercises.

The main characteristic of ancient health care in China is self-massage. It has been widely practiced for at least two thousand years. Records of self-massage can be found in many ancient Chinese writings. In recent years, the traditional Chinese medical experts in scientific research, clinical practice, and medical teaching have further affirmed its practical use.

According to the state of your health, you may want to choose and practice a few of the following exercises. Do them once in the morning and once in the evening. After practicing, close your eyes and rest awhile. Focus your attention on the Dantien (2 cun below the navel) for ten minutes. If you are persistent, you will reap the benefits that you desire.

This exercise is known as *hand-rubbing kung*. (The word *kung* means "exercise.") There are three yin and three yang meridians that run through the human body. Hands are where the yang (Hand-Three-Yang) meridian begins and the yin (Hand-Three-Yin) meridian ends. Therefore, to start taking care of your health, start with your hands. This exercise improves the blood circulation in the hands, making fingers more agile and flexible.

- Put your palms together and rub vigorously until they both feel warm. Rub the back of the right hand with the left hand and rub the back of the left hand with the right hand. Repeat this (left and right) fifteen times.

This one is called *hair-combing kung*. The head is where all meridians meet, so it needs special attention. Practicing hair-combing kung can elevate the yang meridians, so it can refresh you, improve metabolism in the scalp, and prevent or minimize hair loss. In addition, doing this kung routinely will prevent blood rushing to the brain all at once, and at the same time allow adequate blood flow to the brain.

- Instead of using a comb, comb your hair with your ten slightly bent fingers. Move your fingers on your scalp gently back and forth eighty to one hundred times. Then tap your head thoroughly and gently with your fingers for two minutes.

This *eye-rubbing kung* can boost ch'i and keep blood circulating smoothly around the eyes. It will also keep the muscles around the eyes pliable and the eyelids from drooping. In addition, it can also improve eyesight and prevent eye disease.

- Close both eyes. With the soft surface of your middle fingers, rub the lower eyelids from the outer corners of your eyes toward the nose. Rub the upper eyelids from the nose toward the outer corners. Do these massages twenty times each. Then look up, down, left, and right eight times each way.

Teeth-tapping kung can strengthen your teeth. Saliva kills germs and improves digestion. The Chinese in ancient times considered the function of saliva so significant that the character 活 meaning "live" or "alive" was made up of the symbols for water and tongue.

- Every morning after waking up, close your mouth. Tap your teeth thirty-six times. Move your tongue around the gum lines repeatedly so that saliva fills your mouth, then swallow the saliva.

Face-rubbing kung improves blood circulation, minimizes wrinkles, and wards off common colds.

- Rub both hands together until they are warm. Press both palms on the cheekbones with the little fingers pressed close to the sides of the nose. Bring the palms downward to the jaw and back toward the bridge of the nose fifty to a hundred times.

Ear-ringing kung may improve movement of your eardrums and blood circulation in the area ot the ear. It can prevent ringing in the ears and hearing loss. Many functions of the body have corresponding points in the ear area. By rubbing the ears, you are actually improving the health of the entire body.

- Press both ears with your palms. Open and close the ears in an even rhythm six times. With the four fingers (not the thumbs) of both hands, tap the back of your head thirty times. Follow this by rubbing both ears thoroughly thirty times.

Chest-rubbing kung relieves congestion of the chest and symptoms of bronchitis.

- Rub both hands together until they are warm. Rub from the top of the chest downward and back ten times. Then spread out the fingers (like a comb) and rub from the top downward ten times, emphasizing the sides of the chest.

Abdomen-rubbing kung. This kung will improve digestion, prevent bloating and constipation, and even improve your appetite. Release any restraint around the waist before practicing this exercise.

- Rub both hands together until they are warm. Place the left hand on the navel and the right hand on top of the left hand. Rub your abdomen clockwise fifty to one hundred times. The movement should be swift and forceful.

If you do *waist-rubbing kung* persistently, you will enjoy a strong back when you are older. By improving blood circulation it will help keep your kidneys healthy and prevent backache. If you are suffering from backache now, instead of doing this kung eighty-one times, double the number or continue until you are perspiring.

- With both fists, start from the sides of the waist and press the backs of your hands downward to the tailbone and then upward to as far as your arms can reach. Repeat eighty-one times. The movements should be swift and forceful so that your waist feels the heat. While doing this exercise, try to exercise your sphincter muscle by holding and releasing it. Regular exercise of the rectal muscle can prevent hemorrhoids and prostate enlargement.

This next exercise is *foot-rubbing kung*. We all know the importance of our heart's function. Few of us are aware that our feet are the distribution center of various blood vessels and are where the reflex points of most essential organs are located. Traditional Chinese medicine considers the soles of the feet as our "second heart." There are many blood vessels in the foot area. The feet are the farthest away from the heart and therefore blood circulates more slowly there. If you practice this kung once or twice daily to improve blood circulation, you will also indirectly improve the proper function of all major organs and, thereby, your overall health.

Based on research by traditional Chinese medicine, foot rubbing can improve the liver and eyesight, adjust blood pressure, improve sleep, and prevent early aging. It may also help expand the tiny blood vessels of the foot, thereby preventing the numbness and cold and swollen feet that often come with old age.

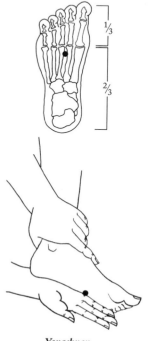

- Rub both hands until they're warm. Touch your left sole with your right hand and the right sole with your left hand. Rub the soles thoroughly one hundred to two hundred times. When rubbing, pay particular attention to the Yongchuan point. The exercise will be more effective if you soak your feet in hot water before going to bed in the evening and then do the foot rubbing. After soaking your feet, thoroughly dry between the toes, then put on moisturizing cream to avoid skin cracks.

Yongchuan

Staying Young

Aging varies with every individual. Some people suffer bad eyesight and shaky teeth before fifty, yet many others maintain good stamina, clear thinking, and good humor into their late eighties and nineties. Why such a disparity? Besides biological reasons, psychological factors play a major role. Therefore, if you would like to stay young, start by thinking youthful thoughts, and follow this advice.

- Think like a youth. Be young at heart. Your mind can help you get healthy and stay healthy. If you can maintain the agile movement and quick thinking of a youth, you can self-stimulate or fool your brain into expanding and working and not realizing that you are aging.
- Train like an athlete. Most athletes train on a systematic and routine basis. To stay young, practice the massages detailed in this book. By exercising regularly you help reduce the chance of your blood vessels being clogged, somethng that happens frequently in the elderly.

- Act like a comedian. When you keep your sense of humor, you not only make others happy, but you also stay young. An authority on aging once said that during a lifetime, our immune system fights a steady battle with enemies of the outer world. But when it turns on its own body, then aging follows. This phenomenon of turning on oneself may be due to years of stress. But if you keep a cheerful and optimistic outlook, you enable your body to produce the substances that combat aging. You also allow your immune system to continually stay on your side.

- Throughout the history of civilization people have searched for the fountain of youth. Before the magic bullet to stop aging is found, try the practice of never overeating. Quit each meal when you are 70–80 percent full. This will be very beneficial to the preservation of your brain function. Also, eat plenty of fruits, vegetables, and juices that are easy to digest and provide plenty of energy and vitality.

8 Patting—To Prevent and Cure Illness

Since ancient times, people throughout the Eastern Hemisphere have held a strong belief that the human body is capable of preventing disease. Ancient Chinese medical experts devised a form of self-treatment that involves patting various parts of the body to promote good health. Patting improves blood circulation and muscle tone, thereby helping our immune systems combat disease when it invades our bodies. Patting is simple and easy.

Head patting can prevent headaches, drowsiness, and other head ailments. At times, minor headaches may disappear or diminish. Since head patting can improve blood circulation in the head and neck, it may also improve memory and clarity of thought.

- Stand erect or sit on a chair. Gaze at whatever is in front of you and relax your entire body. Pat the left side of your head with your left hand and the right side with your right hand. Start with the back of the neck, gradually work up to the forehead, then gradually work your way back.

Repeat this five to eight times.

The *chest and back pat* can boost the respiratory and circulatory systems. With persistent practice, you can also improve your chest and back muscles. You may find it easier to have a partner with whom to do this exercise, since reaching your own back can be awkward.

- Stand erect and relax your entire body. To achieve the best result, wear little or no clothing on your upper body. In a cold climate, it is advisable to do this in a heated room with a thin layer of clothing.

  Hold your hands in loose fists. Pat your right chest with your left hand. Start from the waist and move upward. Do the same with your left chest and right hand. Do two hundred repetitions.

  Pat your right back with the left fist and pat your left back with the right fist. Work from the lower back upward. Do one hundred pats on each side.

The *waist and abdomen pat* will prevent soreness and pains in the waist. It will also relieve symptoms of indigestion, constipation, and bloating. Doing this routinely will make your waist muscles more pliable, thereby avoiding throwing your back out.

- Stand erect and relax your entire body. Pat the waist and abdomen with your fists or fingers as you turn your waist from side to side. For example, when turning to the right, pat the front of your waist and abdomen with your left fist or palm. At the same time, pat your back on the left with the back of your right hand or fist. Pat two hundred times on each side.

The *shoulder pat* can prevent sore shoulder, frozen shoulder, and tendonitis.

- Stand erect or sit straight in a chair. Pat your right shoulder with your left hand and the left shoulder with your right hand, one hundred times for each shoulder.

The *arm pat* can improve the muscle tone of your arms and minimizes any aches and pains resulting from overuse.

- Pat the upper right arm with your left hand and vice versa. Pat thoroughly to ensure the surfaces of both arms are fully covered.

The leg pat prevents numbness and weakness of the legs. For patients that have suffered strokes or lost the use of a leg, the leg pat should improve mobility.

- Sit on a chair, rest your leg on a small stool, and relax. With both hands, pat the leg from top to bottom on all sides two hundred times. Do the same with the right leg.

When patting, relax your entire body. Breathe normally and evenly. Try to focus your thoughts on your body and nothing else. Pat evenly and increase the pressure gradually. Pat in a constant rhythm and cover the entire area. Don't pat randomly. Do it daily at a set time. With the exception of the leg pat, you can walk slowly while patting. The best time to do this exercise is early in the morning. You will feel very relaxed afterward. Do the patting exercise once if it is a preventive measure. Double or triple the patting if an ailment has already developed.

9

A Popular Folk Cure—Gua Sa, or Skin Scraping

Gua sa, or "skin scraping," is a very ancient folk cure that has been widely practiced in China and throughout Asia. Ideally, this should be administered by another person. In some instances, you may be able to do it yourself. I can recall being subjected to this treatment when I was a child living in China. It was almost always in summertime. I can remember that I usually recovered from whatever I was suffering from. The not-so-pleasant memory of someone's scraping my back, neck, or arms lingers.

Recently I had occasion to have this treatment again. This time I was traveling in Taiwan with my husband and my sister. Suddenly I got this nauseated feeling, started to vomit, and experienced severe stomach cramps all at the same time. We were on a bus traveling in the mountains, in the middle of nowhere. An elderly woman in the next seat approached me. Her smile was reassuring. She took a small comb made of animal horn from her hair, and motioned me to lean forward and rest my head on the seat back in front of me. My childhood memories returned and I complied. Skillfully, she started to scrape my back with the comb. My sister, Vivian, was stunned. "Oh, Myrna! Your back is covered with patches of red and purple!" Miraculously, I felt instant relief after the treatment. I sneaked a peak at my fellow passengers behind me and noted gratefully that no one was looking my way. They were either unimpressed or familiar with this procedure.

So what did I have? The Chinese called it *fa sa* or "sand sickness." *Sa,* or "sand," denotes the deep-purple colored, tiny sandlike spots that surface on the skin when the skin is scraped. According to a traditional medicine book: "In the midst of summer or fall, wind, moisture, and heat raise havoc with one's body." Especially when one is exhausted and not accustomed to heat, one is more prone to fa sa, or to feel under the weather. In modern medical terms, this is when one is dehydrated, suffering from heat, and has trouble dispersing the high temperature within one's body effectively.

Fa sa has two significant characteristics. One is that when you start scraping, patches of deep red will surface where there is congestion and remain for a period of time. The other way that you know that you are suffering from fa sa is that you'll get a swollen feeling. Your head, chest, abdomen, and indeed the entire body aches and swells. You will also feel hot and lethargic. In the case of heat-induced fa sa, the symptoms are nausea, dizziness, faintness, palpitations, and lethargy. However, the faces of patients with fa sa caused by lack of air circulation in a closed environment can turn pale and even blue. They may have breathing difficulties and intermittent vomiting. Patients appear incoherent in some cases.

How do you do gua sa? Ideally, the smooth, straight back of a flat comb, preferably made of animal horn or wood, is the best tool. However, a smooth-edged instrument such as a porcelain soup spoon (available in the Chinese grocery store) or a smooth-edged coin will also serve the purpose. Dip the tool in a lubricating salve (such as vegetable oil, olive oil, or water) before you start. Always scrape the skin in one direction, from the top down or from the inside to the outside. Never scrape back and forth. Scrape an area twenty times. Where there is congestion, the skin rapidly discolors and becomes red or purple; this is the desired outcome.

Before you start the scraping treatment, try to place the patient in a cool but not drafty place. The patient should wear loose clothing and either sit or lie down. Start with the patient's back. With firm, deep, long strokes, create two to four lines of patches. Then proceed to the back of the neck. Follow the sides of the neck and then both sides of the chest. Generally, when you have created four to eight lines four to six inches in length, you will have relieved many of the patient's symptoms. If the patient is receptive and feels relief as you're treating him or her, you may scrape one or two more patches next to the spine to maximize the effect of the treatment. In severe cases, when the patient's hands and feet are cold to the touch and muscles are cramping, scrape both arms and the backs of the legs as well.

If the patient is very thin and the backbone is protruding, stay away from the back. Working on the neck will achieve the same effect. Scrape gently on older patients because their skin has less elasticity. Do not scrape off moles, warts, or any other skin irregularities.

During the scraping process, dip your tool in lubricant repeatedly. Never use excess force. You should reassure the patient and get frequent feedback, adjusting your scraping pressure accordingly.

After you have finished the treatment, give the patient a tall glass of water. Add a touch of salt or sugar to stimulate the metabolism.

If no discolored patch is evident in spite of repeated scrapings, and the patient is experiencing symptoms of a cold sweat, vomiting, intermittent diarrhea, or a rapid or weak pulse, stop scraping. Get the patient to a doctor or the hospital emergency room as soon as possible.

Gua sa works, but why? Sometimes when one's body is invaded by unusual weather elements such as wind, cold, heat, and humidity the gland that regulates perspiration shuts down and provides no outlet for the yang ch'i within the body. Skin scraping is an effective way to stimulate, open up, or break up the obstruction of stagnated energy, blood, and fluid. It improves the sluggish circulation and rebalances the yin and yang ch'i, thus relieving the fa sa symptoms. It's simple, easy, and effective.

Acknowledgments

First I want to thank Dr. Ming-sun Yen, who has blind faith in me; Dr. Joseph S. T. Chiang, who patiently reviewed and edited every draft I sent him (and there were many); Mr. Wu Tuan, who brought the original to me and put a bug in my ear; Ms. Katherine Andriessen, who suggested that I take on the challenge; Ms. Irene Tolman, who tirelessly encouraged me to keep going; my dear daughter Mrs. Barbara Han Spitzer, who helped me organize the illustrations while holding her newborn daughter, Siena, with the other hand; Mr. Robert Gillmore, who edited my first draft and provided valuable advice along the way; Mrs. Terri Kelley, who carefully reviewed and corrected my semifinal draft; Mrs. Chris Chen, who made her office machine, supplies, and skills available to me at all times; and Mr. Dee Wang, who helped to put the illustrations onto a disk format. Thank you to acquisitions editor Jon Graham, project editor Susan Davidson, and designer Virginia Scott-Bowman at Healing Arts Press; thank you also to Kam Thye Chow for rendering the final drawings. Last but not least, I want to thank my husband, Michael, who bought me a laptop to do the work on, missed many hot lunches and dinners while I was working on the manuscript, and accompanied me to Fuchow, China, to consult Dr. Yen.

Without you all, this book would never be.